BULLETPROOF
YOUR KNEE

**Optimizing Knee Function to
End Pain and Resist Injury**

by

Jim Johnson, PT

Drawings by Eunice Johnson
Copyright © 2015 Jim Johnson
All Rights Reserved

This edition published by
Dog Ear Publishing
4010 W. 86th Street, Ste H
Indianapolis, IN 46268

www.dogearpublishing.net

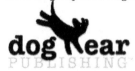
dog Rear
PUBLISHING

ISBN: 978-145754-468-2
Library of Congress Control Number: Applied For
This book is printed on acid-free paper.

Printed in the United States of America

I have given my best effort to ensure that this book is entirely based upon scientific evidence and not on intuition, single case reports, opinions of authorities, anecdotal evidence, or unsystematic clinical observations. Where I do state my opinion in this book, it is directly stated as such.

—*Jim Johnson, P.T.*

WWW.BODYMENDING.COM

TABLE OF CONTENTS

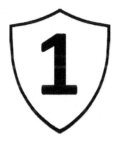

HOW TO BULLETPROOF A KNEE

Having a "bulletproof" knee is just a fun way of saying that you have a knee that is *pain-free* and *resistant to injury*. If you look around, you probably won't have to search too long to find someone with knee pain. Practically everyone has experienced it at one time or another, and for many, it never completely goes away. So just how does one go about "bulletproofing" their knee from pain and injury anyway?

Bulletproofing From Pain

Tackling knee pain is not hard if you go at it with the right approach. Every time someone with knee pain comes to see me, I keep one thought in the back of my mind – the pain is most likely the result of something not functioning properly. My job as a physical therapist, then, is not necessarily to come up with the exact cause of someone's pain, *which can often times be either elusive or controversial*, but rather to figure out what the knee *isn't* doing that it normally should do. Using this approach during my evaluation, I routinely test the various knee functions – such as how strong certain muscles are or how far a patient can bend their knee – so I can then determine what is or is not working up to par. Then, once the improper function has been identified, I can choose an evidence-based treatment that will restore it.

Consider the following list of possible treatments for knee pain...

- hot packs
- arthroscopy

- manual therapy

- total knee replacement

- range-of-motion exercises

- strengthening exercises

- electrical stimulation

- ultrasound

- ice packs

- whirlpool

- exercise bike/treadmill/walking

- massage

- pain medicines

- joint aspiration/injections

As you can see from this rather lengthy list, medicine has come up with quite a wide range of treatment options when it comes to solving the problem of knee pain – and I'm sure there will be many more to come as time goes on.

While at first glance some of them appear to be *very* different from others, they all have a common thread running through them – *each of them is designed to restore or enhance the functioning of the knee area.*

Take a minute and think about it. Ice reduces swelling in your knee so you can bend it easier - and in turn it hurts a lot less. Strengthening exercises provide stability to the knee by making the muscles stronger. The most radical treatment of all, total knee replacement, improves the function of the entire knee area by putting in a new joint that can straighten and flex with ease.

Thinking about treating knee pain in this manner can be quite useful when one is trying to figure out what to do about it. As an example, if a knee is unable to bend as far as it should, then a treatment is needed that will improve the knee's range of motion. And if one of the knee muscles were found to be weak, then a strengthening exercise would be in order. These, then, are the underlying principles this book will use to eliminate any existing knee pain you might have...

Most knee pain is the result of dysfunction. Restore the function with the proper treatment and the pain will be relieved.

Another important point. Having treated knees for over twenty-four years, it's good to be aware of one common pitfall that's easy to fall into when trying to get rid of knee pain – focusing too much on structural abnormalities. What do I mean by *structural abnormalities*?

Well, here I'm talking about things such as bone spurs, worn down or torn cartilage, etc. Now it's not that these kinds of things are insignificant and can't cause pain, *it's just that many people have them and have **no** pain* – so it's best to concentrate on restoring your knee's function first - and then see where you're at. Here are some examples using some common structural abnormalities you've probably heard of, starting with *arthritis*...

- this study looked at 6880 people who had x-rays done of their knees (Hannan 2000). 319 were found to have knee arthritis. Of these 319 subjects, researchers found that 53% had *no pain*. This study shows us that there are many people walking around with knee arthritis that don't hurt.

- yet another interesting x-ray study took 110 men with no knee pain, and x-rayed their knees (Johnson 1998). *41% were found to have bony spurs*, also known as osteophytes, in their knee joints. Remember, these subjects had *no* pain.

- MRI scans have found some pretty interesting things too. Researchers in this study took 49 people with no knee pain and searched for meniscus tears (Bhattacharyya 2003). I'll be going over the knee's structures shortly, but for now, just know that a meniscus is a piece of cartilage - and you have two in each knee. So what did they find? *76% of these subjects with no knee pain had a tear in either their medial or lateral meniscus!* This high percentage is not an isolated finding either - another MRI study found meniscus tears in 63% of pain-free knees (Zanetti 2003)!

Worn down knees, bony spurs, torn cartilage – it's quite amazing that you can find a lot of people walking around with these kind of structural problems, *yet have no pain* - which leaves us a little empty-handed at times trying to explain what exactly causes one's knee pain.

On the other hand though, if you dig into the research on knee pain and *function*, you'll get a little different perspective on things. Here again, by function, I'm talking about how well a knee works and performs. For example, have you ever heard of someone tearing their *ACL*? The ACL or *anterior cruciate ligament* in a very important ligament in your knee that help keeps the knee joint in place (more on that later). Unfortunately, it's also one of the most frequently torn ligaments in your knee – in fact, it gets a lot of abuse in sports such as football.

But as critical as this ligament is to the stability of your knee, wouldn't you think that if *anyone* ruptured their ACL, that they would have a lot of trouble playing a sport, much less walking around? Well, *not exactly*.

Believe it or not, there actually are a significant number of people who have torn their ACL, but are *still* able to use their knees quite well. Here's a quick look at some of the sports medicine literature on this topic...

- more than half of those who rupture their ACL can be classified as *non-copers,* that is they have significant knee instability, even during daily activities, and complain of the knee frequently giving way.

- on the other hand, there are those known as *copers,* who have also ruptured their ACL, but can still maintain high levels of activity. The knee does not give-way, even while doing things such as jumping or pivoting. Furthermore, these lucky individuals are able to return to pre-injury activities without surgery.

- searching to find out why some individuals do remarkably better than others after rupturing their ACL, studies have discovered one important difference – non-copers have *significantly weaker quadriceps muscles* than copers (Eastlack 1999, Eitzen 2010, and Kaplan 2011)

So here we have two groups of people who both have ruptured their ACL's – a *very* important knee ligament. One group (non-copers) experience much knee instability, while the other group (copers) don't. Now if you just looked at the structural abnormalities alone, the torn ligament, you wouldn't be able to tell who had the most knee problems, because both groups have a ruptured ACL. *On the other hand*, if you looked at function (who had the strongest leg muscles), well, you *would* be able to predict who has the most trouble with their knees!

Hmm. Apparently there are *other* problems going on when one has knee pain other than just the structural abnormalities we see pictured all so clearly on MRI's or x-rays – *functional* problems, such as weak muscles should also be taken into consideration.

The point? If you have knee pain, and find you have a torn ligament, arthritis in the joint, or other structural abnormalities such as these, don't panic and feel like all is lost. It is *quite* possible to have a structurally less than perfect knee, yet still feel just fine - so these "normal abnormal findings" might not necessarily be the cause of your pain. That's why it's so important to focus on improving the *function* of your knee first (after seeing a doctor of course), and address any structural abnormalities later on - if ever.

Bulletproofing from Injury

As we talked about earlier, having a bulletproof knee means having a knee that is pain-free and resistant to injury. Getting pain-free is a matter of treating anything that is not functioning properly in your knee and getting it up to par. So what's the plan for becoming resistant to injury?

Well, injury many times involves getting into a situation by chance. One example is falling down. Sometimes we just slip, trip, or twist things – and injure the knee. Other examples are accidents that happen while running or playing a sport.

It's here that there's some good news and some bad news. The bad news is that there's not much you can do about chance occurrences or accidents most of the time – short of "just being careful". The good news, however, is that there is something you can do to eliminate, or at the very least *minimize* your chances of getting hurt when such unlucky events do occur – make sure your knee is *optimally functioning*.

That's right, we're back to the idea of improving knee function again. Just as improving knee function can get rid of pain, it can most certainly build a knee quite resistant to injury. In other words, a knee that has these four abilities can take a lot of abuse…

✓ **Superior Quad Strength**

✓ **Finely-Tuned Control Over the Knee**

✓ **Optimal Flexibility**

✓ **Enhanced Dynamic Knee Stability**

The remainder of this book will go into great detail as to how you can quite easily develop each of the four abilities listed above that are absolutely essential to get a 100% optimally functioning knee, or in other words, a *bulletproof* knee. The diagram on the next page summarizes the concepts that will be used in the chapters that follow...

A normally functioning, pain-free
knee possesses four abilities:

- superior quad strength
- finely-tuned control over the knee
- optimal flexibility
- enhanced dynamic knee stability

Trauma, accidents, and aging changes

Loss of Function

Knee loses one or more of the four abilities:
superior quad strength, finely-tuned control over the knee,
optimal flexibility, enhanced dynamic knee stability

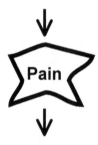

Pain

Regain lost function by doing specific
exercises designed to restore the four abilities

The *Bulletproof* Knee
Pain-free – Resistant to Injury

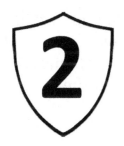

THE PARTS OF YOUR KNEE YOU NEED TO KNOW ABOUT – IN 5 MINUTES

Before you can start bulletproofing your knee, you've got to know what you're dealing with. After all, what mechanic would try to work on a car engine he knew absolutely nothing about? Of course a few readers have probably had that experience before...

Now instead of just listing all the parts of your knee, and then giving you a boring medical definition, we're going to go over the knee's structures by taking a look at pictures of it from the *inside* out. Up first is the basic framework of your knee, *the bones*...

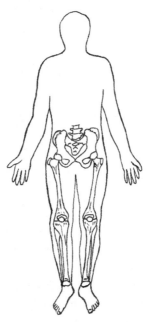

Figure 1. The bones of the upper and lower leg that come together to form your knees.

A look at Figure 1 quickly tells us that the knee is made up of more than just one bone. The following pictures give us a closer look, and reveal to us that the knee is actually made up of three distinct bones; the *femur* (upper leg bone), the *tibia* (the lower leg bone) and the *patella* (your kneecap).

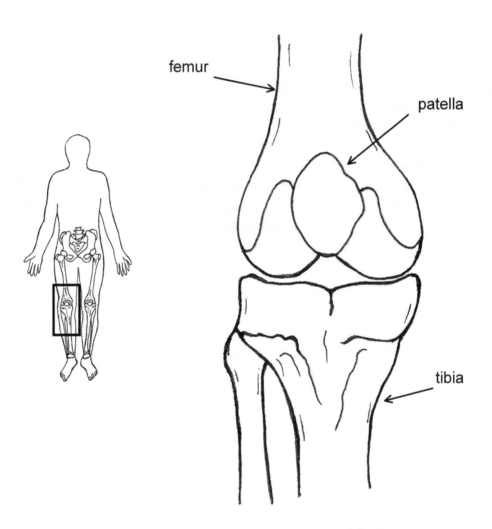

Figure 2. Front view of the three bones that make up the right knee joint.

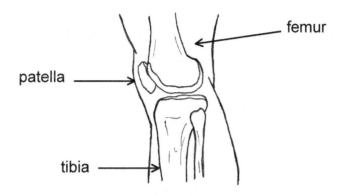

**Figure 3. Side view of the three
bones that make up the knee joint.**

the articular cartilage

Now that you have an idea of what bones make up your knee, it's important to note that where they do come together and meet, their ends are coated with a substance called *articular cartilage.* Being very slick and smooth, it's a big job of the articular cartilage to decrease friction between the bones and help them move smoothly upon one another. Here's a side view showing where the articular cartilage coats the ends of your knee bones...

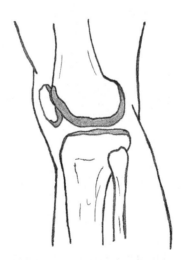

**Figure 4. Shaded areas show where the knee
bones are coated with smooth articular cartilage.**

Here are a few more pictures at different angles. This one is good because it shows the cartilage that is located on the *back* of your knee cap. Yep, you've got cartilage there too!

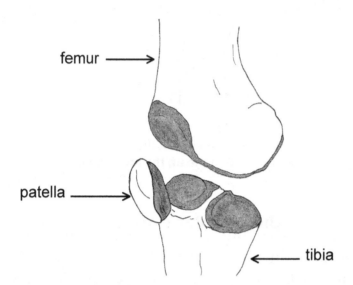

Figure 5. Shaded areas show where the articular cartilage is.

And this one shows the areas of cartilage with the knee cap removed and the knee in a *bent* position.

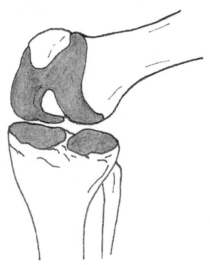

Figure 6. Shaded areas show where the articular cartilage is.

Know that normal articular cartilage is a white, smooth, firm substance that is made up of cells called *chondrocytes*. However unlike other tissues in your body, like the skin or muscles, articular cartilage has *no* blood supply going to it. In other words, there are no small blood vessels going directly to it to provide life-sustaining nutrients. So just how do these tiny little chondrocytes get their nutrition?

To answer that question, we have to take a microscopic look at how the articular cartilage is made up. If you take a piece of articular cartilage from your knee joint, and look at it from the *side* under a powerful microscope, you'd see that it actually has several different layers to it. Check out this picture and you'll see what I mean...

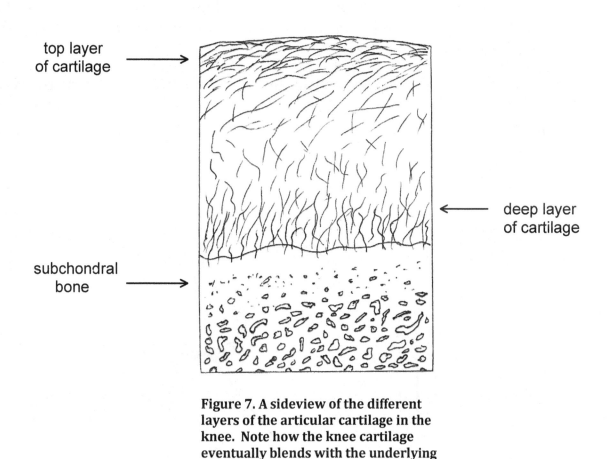

Figure 7. A sideview of the different layers of the articular cartilage in the knee. Note how the knee cartilage eventually blends with the underlying bone.

As you can easily see, there are several different layers to the articular cartilage. Scientists believe that the top layer gets its nutrition from a liquid floating around in the knee joint known as *synovial fluid* (more on that stuff in a few pages).

And the deeper layer of cartilage? It's most likely that it gets its nutrition from the *subchondral bone* it's right next to. In case you're confused, the subchondral bone is just a fancy name for the bone that sits *right under* the layers of cartilage.

the meniscus

Now even though the ends of the tibia and femur are coated with this super-slick articular cartilage stuff that help them move smoothly upon each another, you can see looking back at Figure 6, that the ends of the two bones are shaped *very* differently from each other – not exactly what you'd call "a perfect fit."

So, in order to help this situation, there are two little structures *in between* the two bones called the *medial meniscus*, and *the lateral meniscus.* Pronounced mun-iss-cuss, here's what they look like sitting in your knee...

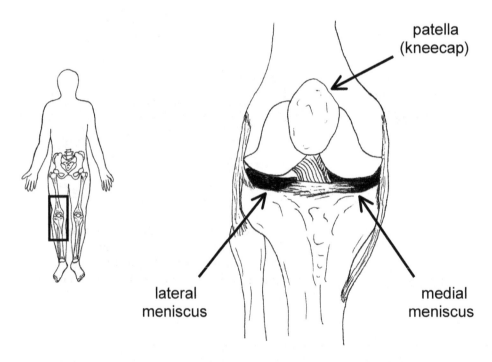

patella
(kneecap)

lateral
meniscus

medial
meniscus

**Figure 8. Front view of the medial
and lateral meniscus of the right knee.**

Since the upper bone of the knee, the femur, has two *round* parts that sit directly on the *flatter* tibia bone, you can see how the medial and lateral meniscus really help improve the fit between the two bones.

Now that you've seen what the medial and lateral meniscus look like from the front, let's lift up the femur a bit to get a better look at things...

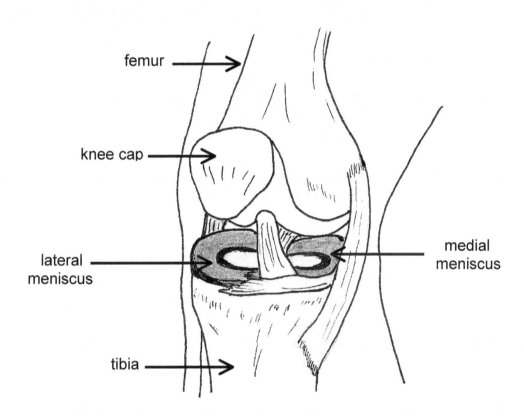

Figure 9. How the medial and lateral meniscus sit in the right knee joint.

Like the articular cartilage that coats the end of the bones, the medial and lateral meniscus are also made of cartilage, however it's a different kind called *fibrocartilage*.

Besides helping the femur and tibia fit together a little better, the medial and lateral meniscus also help out with shock absorption and work hard to transmit forces across the knee more efficiently. This last picture reveals how different the medial and lateral meniscus really are in shape...

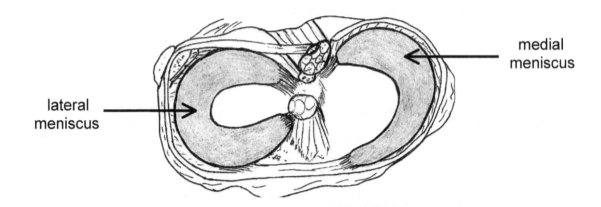

lateral
meniscus

medial
meniscus

**Figure 10. Overhead view of the
medial and lateral meniscus.**

the ligaments

Okay. Up to this point we've got two bones covered with smooth articular cartilage on their ends, that are neatly fitted together with two pieces of fibrocartilage in between them. So the next question is, what *keeps* them together? Well, it's a specialized connective tissue known as a *ligament*.

While there are many different ligaments in and around the knee, some big, some small, we're going to take a look at the major ones. There are four of them, and they are:

- the anterior cruciate ligament

- the posterior cruciate ligament

- the medial collateral ligament

- the lateral collateral ligament

Since it's the job of the ligaments to hold the bones together, it's logical that they'd have to run from one bone to another. Let's see exactly where they are in the knee...

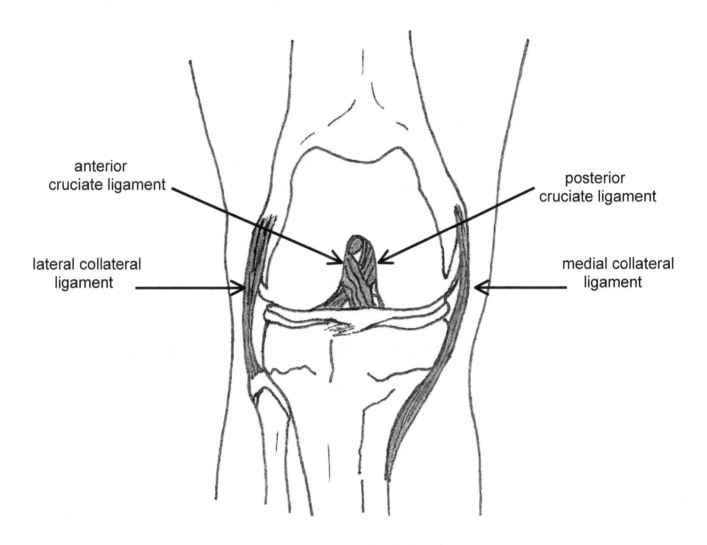

anterior
cruciate ligament

posterior
cruciate ligament

lateral collateral
ligament

medial collateral
ligament

Figure 11. Front view of the four major ligaments of the right knee that help hold the bones in place.

Did you notice that the two ligaments in the middle cross each other and make an "x"? That's why they were named the *cruciate* ligaments, because "cruciate" comes from the Latin word "crux" – which means cross. By the way, if you've ever heard of an athlete tearing their "ACL", it was the **A**nterior **C**ruciate **L**igament that they tore. Ouch!

While these four ligaments work hard all day to help hold your knee bones in place, don't think that they just sit there stiff as a board. If that was the case, you wouldn't be able to move your knee around very much!

So just how do these ligaments work? Well, a ligament will allow a certain amount of motion to take place in the knee, but, if a bone starts going *too far* in one direction, growing tension in the ligament stops it. By working this way, the ligaments can both *permit* a certain amount of knee motion, as well as *limit* it. Take a look at these examples and you'll see how the ligaments react as you move your knee around…

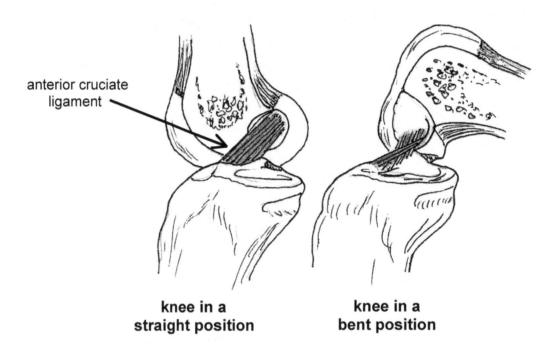

anterior cruciate
ligament

**knee in a
straight position**

**knee in a
bent position**

**Figure 12. A side view showing how the
anterior cruciate ligament reacts when
you bend and straighten your knee.**

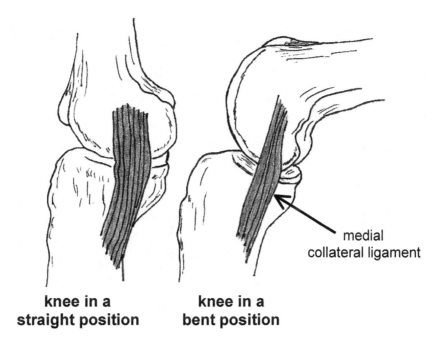

**knee in a
straight position**   **knee in a
bent position**

**Figure 13. A side view showing how the
medial collateral ligament reacts when
you bend and straighten your knee.**

the synovial membrane

I doubt a lot of readers have heard of this knee structure. The *synovial membrane* is like a "sleeve" that fits neatly around your knee joint and envelopes it. This is what it looks like :

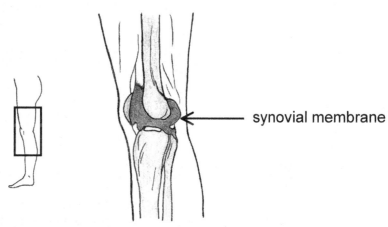

Figure 14. The synovial membrane

Interesting structure, isn't it? Think of the synovial membrane kind of like a plastic wrap that clings closely to the entire knee joint. Here are a few more pictures to give you a better look...

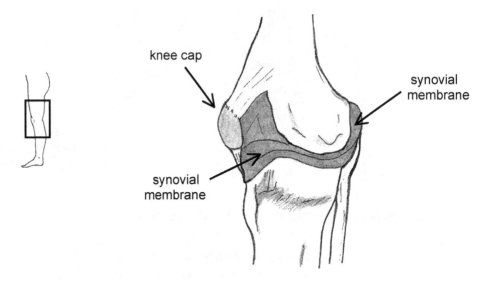

Figure 15. A side view of the synovial membrane

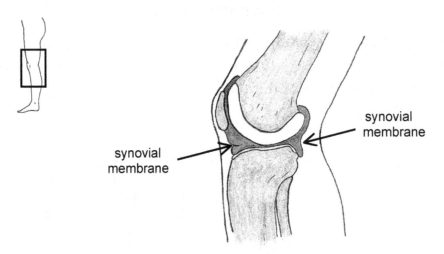

Figure 16. A cut-out side view of the synovial membrane. Note how the synovium wraps itself around the two bones and "seals in" the knee joint.

So what does the synovial membrane do? Well, it lines the joint and makes that substance we talked about on page 14 called *synovial fluid*. Synovial fluid is a must-have to your knee, because it floats around and provides nutrients to the cartilage in your knee. Additionally, it also helps lubricate your knee joint.

the bursae

Have you ever heard of bursitis? A lot of people have. It's common in the shoulder, and you get it when you have a problem with a small structure called a *bursae* (pronounced burr-sah). So what's a bursae?

Well, bursae in general are flat, sac-like structures that are located *all* throughout your body. If you've ever seen a deflated whoopie cushion, well, that's about what they look like. It's the main job of these bursae to reduce friction and make things slide a whole lot easier, particularly in areas where structures have a tendency to rub together a lot – like where a tendon passes right over a bone.

Now normally these little guys contain a small amount of fluid, however if they get really irritated for any number of reason, well, they can really swell up and cause you a lot of pain – and then you've got bursitis. You've got a bunch of bursae around your knee joint, and here's a picture of some of the major ones...

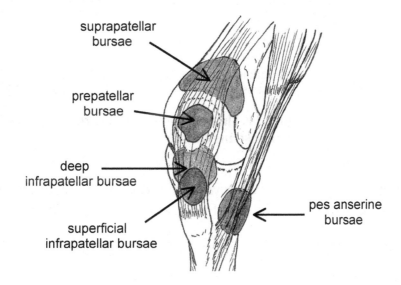

suprapatellar
bursae

prepatellar
bursae

deep
infrapatellar bursae

superficial
infrapatellar bursae

pes anserine
bursae

**Figure 17. Some of the major
bursae around the right knee.**

the muscles

Well, we're finally to the last and outermost structure of your knee, the muscles, which make your knee move. While there are quite a few of them in and around the knee, I just want you to be familiar with two major groups in particular – the *quadriceps* and the *hamstrings*. As the following pictures show, the quadriceps muscles take up most of the *front* of your thigh, while the hamstrings make up most of the *back*. Here's a look at where they are...

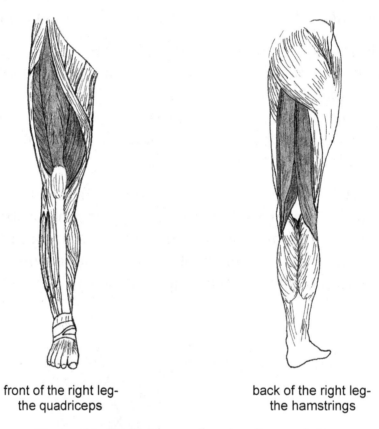

front of the right leg-
the quadriceps

back of the right leg-
the hamstrings

Figure 18. Shaded areas showing the quadriceps and hamstring muscle groups.

And that's it – a quick overview of the key knee structures you'll need to know about in order to bulletproof your knee. Next up, *Step 1...*

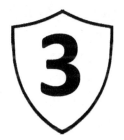

STEP ONE: KEEP YOUR QUADS STRONG

It would be quite hard for you to do much at all without the help of your muscles. Even something as basic and simple as walking requires the forces from no fewer than *twenty-eight* of your leg muscles in order for you to carefully control the pull of gravity as you try to move forward. As you can see, muscles act as "engines" that your body uses to make itself move. The following is a list of some of the muscles that are situated in and around the knee area...

- sartorius

- gracilis

- adductor magnus and longus

- the quadriceps – vastus lateralis, medialis, intermedius, and rectus femoris

- the hamstrings – semimembranosus, semitendinosus, and biceps femoris

- gastrocnemius

- popliteus

As you can see, there are many leg muscles with unusual names. They all play a part, one way or another, in the functioning of our knees. However, many studies over the years have pointed out that some of these muscles clearly deserve more attention than others when it comes to knee problems. It appears as though some muscles, for various reasons, are "hit harder" when you have a problem with your knee. Strangely enough, some muscles are able to continue working adequately in the face of swelling or sudden injury to the knee, while others respond by getting weaker or smaller, or by shutting down altogether. For the purposes of this book, you can take this as really good news. It means that you will not have to spend a lot of time doing countless exercises to strengthen each of the individual muscles in the knee area.

A Selective Problem

Over the years, I have spent a great deal of time in the medical library, trying to find out exactly what knee conditions affect which muscles. When I initially started my investigation in this area, I expected the research to show, for example, that arthritis caused problems mainly for one or two muscles, while a torn ligament took its toll on a completely different muscle. What I found, however, was rather surprising. It quickly became apparent that for just about every single knee condition I was checking out (such as arthritis, ligament tears, etc.) *the same muscle* kept cropping up over and over as being the one most affected. And just what muscle was it?

In the cadaver lab, back in physical therapy school, we learned the muscle's Latin name, *musculus quadriceps femoris*. Most doctors and physical therapists, however, commonly call it the *quadriceps*, which literally translates into "four-headed muscle." If you're like me, and prefer nicknames, you can just call it "the quads."

The quads are indeed made up of four distinct muscles. They are the following...

- ✓ vastus lateralis
- ✓ vastus medialis
- ✓ vastus intermedius
- ✓ rectus femoris

The first three muscles, the vastus lateralis, vastus medialis, and vastus intermedius, all attach themselves to the bone of your upper leg, cross your knee in front, and then attach to the big bone in your lower leg. The last one, rectus femoris, attaches itself a little bit differently. It starts out at your hip area, just below your belt line in the front, and then continues down to cross your knee like the other three vastus muscles.

Figure 19 is a close-up illustration of the quads, looking at the right leg from the front. Note that you can only see three of the four muscles of the quadriceps, as the vastus intermedius lies neatly buried under the rectus femoris.

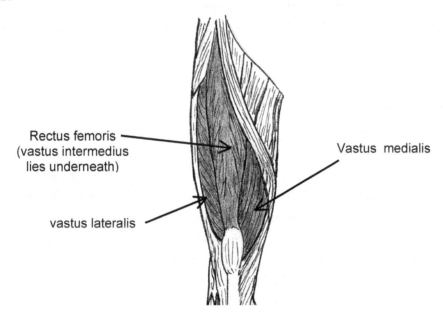

Figure 19. The quadriceps muscle group, also known as "the quadriceps" or "the quads".

So just what do the quads do? Well, if you're sitting in a chair at the moment, kick out your leg. This action is one of the main job of the quads, that is, they help you straighten out your leg. Now try this. Stand up from a sitting position, and as you do so, put one hand onto the front of your thigh. You should be able to feel the muscles under your hand (the quads) tighten and firm up as you begin to rise. This is yet another important function of this muscle. With your foot fixed on the floor as you stand up, the quads work to pull you into a standing position. Along with these activities, your quads are also largely responsible for your ability to walk, run, jump, and climb stairs. Additionally, the knee joint itself depends heavily on the quads to help stabilize and support it. *As you will soon see, knee problems tend to cause isolated muscle wasting and weakness, specifically in the quadriceps group – making this a key muscle to keep in shape when bulletproofing a knee.*

Effects of Various Knee Problems on the Quads

Let's take a brief look now at the evidence from peer-reviewed journals that have shown the quadriceps to be affected by a variety of knee conditions. (Peer-reviewed journals are magazines that only publish articles that have been reviewed by experts in the field.)

Knee Swelling and the Quadriceps

Experiencing swelling in your knee has been shown to be a major reason why your quads might not be working like they should. If you were to lie flat on your back as I injected a harmless salt-water solution known as *saline* into your knee, you would find that after a certain amount of this fluid entered your knee joint, you would no longer be able to lift your leg off the table. Then, as I removed the saline a little at a time, you would slowly start to regain control of your leg once again – and be able to lift it. Here's what some of the studies that have looked into this unusual effect of having extra fluid in the knee joint have found...

- one study took patients with chronic (long-term) knee swelling, removed the excess fluid using a needle, and amazingly measured an *immediate increase* in quadriceps strength (Fahrer 1988)

- another study demonstrated that even if you have as little as 20 milliliters of fluid in your knee (which is just over a tablespoon), it's enough to *decrease* the strength of your quadriceps muscle (Spencer 1984)

- this interesting experiment took subjects with no knee problems, and measured their quadriceps strength after 60 milliliters of saline was injected in their knee joint – 20 milliliters at a time (Jensen 1993). Investigators found that quadriceps strength *decreased* as more and more saline was injected. Likewise, quadriceps strength increased as the saline was removed.

As you can see, it takes a whole lot less than a huge, swollen knee in order to prevent your quadriceps muscle from working properly. According to the research, having just over a tablespoon of fluid in the knee – probably too small an amount for most people to visibly notice – is sufficient to trigger a problem.

Knee Injuries and the Quadriceps

Studies have also taken a close look at how the muscles of the leg respond to a knee injury. For instance…

- sixteen people who had *recently* fallen on their knee, or sustained a direct blow to their kneecap, were examined (Manal 2000)

- testing revealed that only 69% of subjects were able to fully activate their quadriceps – leaving one-third with problems!

Along the same lines, the quadriceps muscle of people with *a history* of knee injury has also been examined in detail. By using an ultrasound machine, pictures could be taken of the individual leg muscles, and the size of each one could be assessed (Young 1980). Subjects in this study had a wide range of diagnoses, including...

- surgical removal of part of the knee cartilage

- various knee injuries

- fractured tibia (a lower leg bone)

- surgical opening of the knee joint

- pes anserine (tendon) transfer

Additionally, each subject had their mid-thigh circumference measured with a tape measure to detect any size differences between legs. As one would expect, in most cases, the injured leg was smaller around than the non-injured leg, possible indicating that some of the muscles had wasted away due to injury. The exact muscles involved, however, could not be determined with a simple tape-measurement technique. It took the aid of the ultrasound picture for the researchers to accurately tell that the muscle wasting process was largely due to just one muscle – the quadriceps!

Ligament Problems and the Quadriceps

As we touched on briefly in the last chapter, ligaments are tough fibrous tissues that attach bones to each other – making one of their primary functions to help stabilize the joints. As you can probably guess, problems with ligaments in the knee can also spell trouble for the quadriceps muscle. Looking back at Figure 11 on page seventeen, you can see the major ligaments in the knee. Let's take a brief look at what the research says about how injuring some of them can affect the quadriceps muscle...

the anterior cruciate ligament

We talked a little about this ligament on pages 17 and 18. Known most popularly as "the ACL", the anterior cruciate ligament controls motion between the lower leg bone, the tibia, and the upper leg bone, the femur. A lot of anterior cruciate ligament injuries occur when the knee is forcefully twisted or hyperextended (bent backwards) – which can tear and even rupture this ligament. If the rip is severe enough, the knee joint can eventually become unstable, leading to what most orthopedic surgeons refer to as "instability". Not good news for the quadriceps muscle either…

- one study looked at people who had *completely* ruptured their ACL, and were scheduled for surgical reconstruction (Hsiao 2014). *Researchers found that the strength of their quadriceps muscle in the injured leg was decreased by 25 to 30%.*

- it doesn't look good over the long run either. One study followed subjects with complete ACL ruptures (who had no surgery) for a whopping 15 years – and found that only 75% of them had normal quad strength (Ageberg 2007).

the posterior cruciate ligament

Like the ACL, the posterior cruciate ligament (or PCL) also helps control the motion between the tibia and femur – but fortunately gets injured much less frequently. But when it does, a similar thing happen to your quads…

- 20 patients with isolated tears of their PCL, all candidates for reconstructive surgery, were tested (Lee 2015). *Results showed a significant decrease in quad strength in the injured leg.*

- long-term follow-up studies on PCL injuries show similar results (Tibone 1988). One study followed a group of 10 untreated patients with a ruptured PCL for six years. What did they find? *The injured knee still had a 20% decrease in quad strength.*

the medial collateral ligament

In addition to the anterior and posterior cruciate ligament, the medial collateral ligament (MCL) has also been investigated. As seen in Figure 11 (page 17), this ligament is located along the inner part of your knee, and sits vertically across the joint – rather like a piece of tape holding the two leg bones together. Its job is to prevent the knee from buckling inward, and it is commonly injured when a force is applied to the outside of the knee, as in a football clipping injury. And when it does get injured, guess what happens to your quads...

- researchers investigated a group of subjects with medial collateral ligament injuries (Kannus 1988)

- 54 had partial tears, and 27 had complete tears

- they were followed for an average of 9 years after the injury, at which time they had the strength of their quadriceps muscles tested

- interestingly, those that had partial tears years ago showed a 4% quadriceps strength deficit, while those that had *complete* tears showed a whopping 21% quad deficit. More recent studies have also shown long-standing quadriceps weakness after an MCL tear (Al-Hourani 2015).

Knee Pain and the Quadriceps

Riann Palmieri-Smith and colleagues at the University of Michigan conducted an interesting study that illustrates just how effectively pain can cause a major loss of quadriceps strength...

- 14 men and women with healthy knees participated in this study (Palmieri-Smith 2013)

- in one of the experimental conditions, these subjects had a substance injected into their knee to irritate the joint and cause pain (ouch).

- the strength of the quadriceps muscle was tested before *and* after the injection that caused knee pain

- researchers were able to show that the knee pain actually caused a *14% decrease* in quadriceps strength

So as you can see, it doesn't even take a direct injury – just having pain in your knee can give you significant weakness of a key muscle that supports and stabilizes it!

Knee Arthritis and the Quadriceps

Arthritis – or more specifically osteoarthritis – of the knee has taken its place as one of the most common causes of chronic disability among the elderly. I have treated many patients for it, and am willing to bet that some readers of this book have been diagnosed with it.

Since this condition is so widespread, you may have guessed that an enormous amount of research has been published on the topic. In order to give you all the "important stuff", without getting too bogged down in piles of research, I have chosen to summarize the information you most need to be aware of. It is as follows...

- 54 people with symptomatic knee osteoarthritis were compared to 43 controls with normal knees matched for age and sex (Liikavainio 2008). This means that if you are a 50 year-old woman with knee arthritis, your knees were compared to another 50 year-old woman with normal knees. Comparisons of these two groups revealed that the people with knee osteoarthritis had 20% weaker quad muscles than those with normal knees.

- another study (Hurley 1993) looked at people who had osteoarthritis in just one knee. After strength testing, it was found that the quadriceps muscle in the arthritic knee was 40 percent weaker than in their normal knee.

- some readers may be thinking that perhaps people with knee osteoarthritis show muscle weakness in all these studies simply because it hurts when they move their knee, thus preventing them from showing their true strength. A good thought, however when researchers study random groups of people using x-rays and strength tests, quadriceps weakness also exists in persons with knee osteoarthritis who have no knee pain (Slemenda 1997).

As you can see, it is well established in the medical literature that the quadriceps muscle is clearly affected when it comes to knee osteoarthritis.

One last thing to be aware of. Recently, a group of researchers conducted a systematic review of the published literature looking into the link between having weak quadriceps muscles, and getting knee osteoarthritis (Oiestad 2015). What did they find? Well, when they finished sifting through the entire scientific literature, they concluded that the evidence showed that *quadriceps muscle weakness was associated with an increased risk of developing knee osteoarthritis in both men and women!* Which gives us just *one more* reason to keep our quads in good shape to stay out of trouble...

Patellofemoral Pain Syndrome and the Quadriceps

Have you ever heard of *patellofemoral pain syndrome*? Most people haven't, and don't know much about it until they get it. When this happens, a person usually complains of pain under or around the kneecap – which is often aggravated when the knee is bent (squatting, going up stairs, etc). This is the last major knee condition I know of that takes a significant toll on the quadriceps muscle...

- researchers in this study looked at 24 women with patellofemoral pain syndrome in one knee (Kaya 2011). MRI images were taken of their leg muscles, and the strength of their quadriceps muscles were tested. When results were compared to their healthy knee, MRI images showed that the knee with patellofemoral pain syndrome had a much smaller quadriceps muscle – and strength testing showed it to be much weaker too.

- along the same lines, another study took 46 patients with patellofemoral pain syndrome and compared them to 30 age and sex matched control subjects with healthy knees (Pattyn 2011). MRI images showed that those with patellofemoral pain syndrome had a much *smaller* quadriceps muscle.

Seems like a broken record, doesn't it? Yet again, we have another knee condition that is associated with weak quadriceps. And when all is said and done, we have quite a big list...

The following conditions have been associated with muscle wasting and weakness in the quadriceps:

- ✓ **swelling in the knee**

- ✓ **having had surgery on the knee**

- ✓ **history of injuries, including falls or direct blows to the knee**

- ✓ **fractures of the tibia**

- ✓ **having torn knee ligaments**

- ✓ **having knee pain**

- ✓ **having arthritis in the knee**

- ✓ **having patellofemoral pain syndrome**

Surefire Ways to Strengthen Your Quadriceps Muscle

Okay, enough research for now. Since we know that the majority of knee problems are linked to weak quads, the next step is to improve knee function – and make it *stronger.*

However before jumping right in and going over all the exercises you'll ever need to beef up your quadriceps, I think it's best to begin with a few strength training basics. Because I wrote this book with *everyone* in mind – from the athlete, to the retired person who just wants to be able to walk with their grandkids – it's only wise to make sure that we're all on the same page before going any further. Then, when we do get down to describing each of the strengthening exercises, *every* reader will know exactly what I mean when I say, "Do 1 set of 20 reps." So, using the handy question and answer format, let's start with the basics...

How do we make a muscle stronger?

Muscles get stronger only when we constantly challenge them to do more than they're used to doing. Do the same amount and type of activity over and over again, and your muscles will *never* increase in strength. For example, if Karen goes to the gym and lifts a ten-pound dumbbell up and down, ten times, workout after workout, week after week, her arms will *not* get any stronger by doing this exercise. Why? Because the human body is very efficient.

You see, right now, Karen's arm muscles can already do the job she is asking them to do (lift a ten-pound dumbbell ten times). Therefore, why should they bother growing any stronger? I mean after all, stronger, bigger muscles *do* require more calories, nutrition and maintenance from the body. And since they can *already* do everything they're asked to do, increasing in size and demanding more from the rest of the body would only be a waste of resources for no good reason.

It makes perfect sense if you stop and think about it, but we can also use this same line of thinking when it comes to making our muscles bigger and stronger – we simply *give* them a reason to get into better shape. And how do we do that? By simply asking them to do *more* than they're used to doing. Going back to the above example, if Karen wants make her arm muscles stronger, then she could maybe switch from a ten-pound dumbbell to a *twelve*-pound dumbbell the next time she goes to work out. Whoa! Her arm muscles won't be ready for that at all – they were always used to working with that ten-pound dumbbell. And so, they will have no choice but to get stronger now in order to meet the *new* demand Karen has placed on them.

For the more scientific-minded readers, the physiology textbooks call this *progressive resistance exercise.* You can use this very same strategy to get *any* muscle in your body stronger, and we're certainly going to be using it to get our quads as strong as we can.

What's the difference between a repetition and a set?

As we've said, we need to constantly challenge our muscles in order to force them to get stronger, and one good way to do this is to lift a little heavier weight than we're used to using. Of course you won't always be able to lift a heavier and heavier weight *every* time you do an exercise, and so another option you have is to try to lift the same weight *more* times than you did before. As you can see, it's a good idea to keep track of things, just so you know for sure that you're actually making progress – which is where the terms "set" and "repetition" come into play.

If you take a weight and lift it up and down over your head once, you could say that you have just done one repetition or "rep" of that exercise. Likewise, if you take the same weight and lift it up and down a total of ten times over your head, then you could say that you did ten repetitions of that exercise.

A set, on the other hand, is simply a bunch of repetitions done one after the other. Using our above example once again, if you lifted a weight ten times over your head, and then rested, you would have just done one set of ten repetitions. Pretty straightforward isn't it?

Now the last thing you need to know about reps and sets is how we go about writing them down. The most common method used, is to first write the number of sets you did of an exercise, followed by an "x", and then the number of repetitions you did. For example, if you were able to lift a weight over your head ten times and then rested, you would write down 1x10. This means that you did 1 set of 10 repetitions of that particular exercise. Likewise, if the next workout you did 12 repetitions, you would write 1x12.

What's the best number of sets and repetitions to do in order to make a muscle stronger?

There was a time when I asked myself that same question. So, in order to find out, I completely searched the published strength training literature starting from the year 1960. I then sorted out just the randomized controlled trials, since these provide the highest form of proof in medicine that something is really effective, and laid them all out on my kitchen table. While getting to that point took me literally months and months of daily reading and hunting down articles, it was really the only way I could come up with an accurate, evidence-based answer.

Now the first conclusion I came to, was that it is quite possible for a person to get significantly stronger by doing any one of a *wide* variety of set and repetition combinations. For instance, one study might show that one set of eight to twelve repetitions could make a person stronger compared to a non-exercising control group – but then again so could four sets of thirteen to fifteen reps in another study.

Realizing this, I decided to change my strategy a bit and set my sights on finding the most *efficient* number of sets and repetitions. In other words, how many sets and repetitions could produce the *best* strength gains with the *least* amount of effort? And so, I had two issues to resolve. The first one was, "Are multiple sets of an exercise better than doing just one set?" and the second, "Exactly how many repetitions will produce the best strength gains?"

Anxious to get to the bottom of things, I returned once again to my pile of randomized controlled trials, this time searching for more specific answers. Here's what I found as far as sets are concerned:

- there are *many* randomized controlled trials showing that *one* set of an exercise is **just as good** as doing *three* sets of an exercise (Esquivel 2007, Starkey 1996, Reid 1987, Stowers 1983, Silvester 1982). This has been shown to be true in people who have just started weight training, as well in individuals that have been training for some time (Hass 2000).

Wow. With a lot of my patients either having limited time to exercise, or just plain hating it altogether, that was really good news. I could now tell them that based on strong evidence from many randomized controlled trials, all they needed to do was just *one set* of an exercise to get stronger – which would get them every bit as strong as doing three!

And the best number of repetitions to do? Well, that wasn't quite as cut and dried. The first thing I noted from the literature was that different numbers of repetitions have totally different training effects on the muscles. You see, it seems that the lower numbers of repetitions, say three or seven for example, train the muscles more for *strength*. On the other hand, the higher repetition numbers, such as twenty or twenty-five, tend to increase a muscle's *endurance* more than strength (endurance is where a muscle must repeatedly contract over and over for a long period of time, such as when a person continuously moves their arms back and forth while vacuuming a rug for several minutes).

Another way to think about this is to simply imagine the repetition numbers sitting on a line. Repetitions that develop *strength* sit more toward the far left side of the line, and the number of repetitions that develop mainly *endurance* lie towards the right. Everything in the middle, therefore, would give you varying mixtures of both strength *and* endurance. The following is an example of this:

The Repetition Continuum

1 rep	10 reps	around 20 reps and higher

strength ————————————— endurance ————————→

Please note, however, that it's not like you won't gain *any* strength at all if you do an exercise for twenty repetitions or more. It's just that you'll gain mainly muscular endurance, and not near as much strength than if you would have done fewer repetitions (such as five or ten).

Okay, so now I knew there was a big difference between the lower repetitions and the higher repetitions. However one last question still stuck in my mind. Among the lower repetitions, are some better than others for gaining strength? For example, can I tell my patients that they will get stronger by doing a set of three or four repetitions as opposed to doing a set of nine or ten?

Well, it turns out that there really is no difference. For example, one randomized controlled trial had groups of exercisers do either three sets of 2-3 repetitions, three sets of 5-6 repetitions, or three sets of 9-10 repetitions (O'Shea 1966). After six weeks of training, everyone improved in strength, *with no significant differences among the three groups.*

And so, with this last piece of information, my lengthy (but profitable) investigation had finally come to an end. After scrutinizing some 45-plus years of strength training research, I could now make the following evidence-based conclusions...

✓ doing one set of an exercise is just as good as doing three sets of an exercise
✓ lower repetitions are best for building muscular strength, with no particular lower number being better than the others
✓ higher repetitions (around 20 or more) are best for building muscular *endurance*

In this book, we'll be taking full advantage of the above information by doing just one set of an exercise for ten to twenty repetitions. This means that you will use a weight that you can lift *at least* ten times in a row, and when you can lift it twenty times in good form, it's time to increase the weight a little to keep the progress going.

And why did I pick those numbers? Two reasons. The first has to do with the job of the quadriceps muscle. Since it plays a big role in stabilizing your knee, we want to increase its endurance and long holding time the most – so this means we're going to lean a little more towards the *upper* repetitions in order to boost the endurance ability of the quadriceps – while still staying low enough to substantially increase its strength. Remember, from around the twenty repetitions mark and up, you're going to gain mostly muscular endurance, and a lot less strength.

The second reason? Well, it's a matter of safety. Using higher repetitions enables us to not only gain plenty of strength, but also use much *lighter* weights than if we'd chosen to work with the lower repetitions. This is because it takes a much heavier weight to tire a muscle out in, say, five repetitions, than it does to tire a muscle out in fifteen. And since most people would agree that you have a better chance of injuring yourself with a heavier weight as opposed to a lighter one, I recommend leaning more towards the *upper* repetitions.

How many times a week do I have to do a strengthening exercise?

Doing the same strengthening exercise every day, or even five days a week, will usually lead to overtraining – which means *no* strength gains. This is because the muscles need time to recover, which typically means at least a day or so in between exercise bouts to rest and rebuild before you stress 'em again. And so, the question then becomes, which is better, one, two or three times a week?

Well, believe it or not, when I went through the strength training literature in search of the optimal number of times a week to do a strengthening exercise, there were a few randomized controlled trials actually showing that doing a strengthening exercise *once* a week was just as good as doing it two or three times a week. However, these studies were done on *very* specific populations (such as the elderly) or *very* specific muscle groups that were worked in a special manner. Therefore, when you take this information, and couple it with the fact that there are a few randomized controlled trials showing that two and three times a week are far better than one time a week, there really isn't much support for the average person to do a strengthening exercise once a week to get stronger. And so, we're again left with another question of which is better, two versus three times a week–which is what much of the strength training research has investigated.

However it is at this point that the waters start to get a little muddy. If you take all the randomized controlled trials comparing two times a week to three times a week, and lay them out on a table, you will get mixed results. In other words, there are some studies showing you that doing an exercise two times a week will get you the *same* results as three times a week, **but** there's also good research showing you that three times a week is *better* than two times a week. So what's one to do?

Well, in a case like this, the bottom line is that you can't really draw a firm conclusion one way or the other. So, you've got to work with what you've got. In this book, I'm going to recommend that you shoot for doing the strengthening exercises *three* times a week, because there is some good evidence that three times a week is better than two times a week (Braith 1989). However, I'm also going to add that if you have an unbelievably busy week, or just plain forget to do the exercises, I'll settle for two times a week because there is also substantial evidence that working out two times a week is just as good as working out three times a week (Carroll 1998, DeMichele 1997).

So there you have it. While it may have been a whole lot easier to just answer the question by saying "do the strengthening exercise two to three times a week," I think it's good for readers to know *exactly* why they're doing the things I'm suggesting *and* that there's a good, evidence-based reason behind it.

How hard should I push it when I do a set?

How hard you push yourself while doing an exercise, also known as *exercise intensity*, is another issue that certainly deserves mention and is a question I am frequently asked by patients. The answer lies in two important pieces of information:

1. Doing an exercise until no further repetitions can be done in good form is called *momentary muscular failure*. Research shows us that getting to momentary muscular failure, or close to it, produces the best strength gains.

2. You should not be in pain while exercising.

Taking the above information into consideration, I feel that a person should keep doing an exercise as long as it isn't painful and until no further repetitions can be done in good form within the repetition scheme.

Does it make any difference how fast you do a repetition?

Many randomized controlled trials have shown that as far as gaining strength is concerned, it does *not* matter whether you do a repetition fast or slow (Berger 1966, Palmieri 1987, Young 1993). Here's a look at one of the studies:

- subjects were randomly divided into three groups (Berger 1966)

- each group did one set of the bench press exercise, which was performed in 25 seconds

- the first group did 4 repetitions in 25 seconds, the second group did 8-10 repetitions in 25 seconds, and the third did 18-20 repetitions in 25 seconds

- at the end of eight weeks, *there were no significant differences in the amount of strength gained between any of the groups*

So that's the evidence-based guidelines as far as strength is concerned. As far as safety, I recommend that you lift the weight up and down *smoothly* with each repetition, carefully avoiding any jerking motions.

What equipment will I need?

Since you'll be doing a strengthening exercise that involves lifting weights, it's a no brainer you're going to need something to lift. Remember from our discussion on pages 34 and 35 that muscles get stronger only when we constantly challenge them to do more than they're used to doing. So, this means that taking the same weight, and lifting it over and over again, week after week, simply won't get the job done. Therefore, you'll need to have *several* weights of varying pounds available to use.

Now if you think this will involve a lot of money, it doesn't have to. By far, the easiest and cheapest way to go is to buy a set of *adjustable* ankle weights. You can get them at most sporting good stores and they typically look something like this:

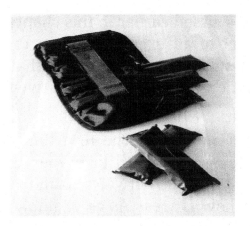

As you can see from the picture, the cuff can attach quite easily to your ankle by means of a velcro strap. Also note that the cuff is made up of six mini weight packs that you can take in and out of their little pockets, depending on how many pounds you want to use. Since the cuff in the picture weighs a total of 10 pounds, and has six little packs, this means that each one weighs a little over a pound and a half. This allows you to increase the weight *gradually* on any given exercise – which is one of the biggest advantages of using *adjustable* cuff weights.

Some tips on buying them. First, be aware that there are *wrist* cuffs and there are *ankle* cuffs (the above picture shows an ankle cuff). Wrist cuffs are smaller, but I recommend getting the ankle cuffs, mainly because they are heavier which allows you to go up higher in weight over time than the wrist cuffs. Second, pay particular attention to how many total pounds *each cuff* weighs. How much weight should you look for? Probably two 10-pound cuffs will give you a good workout for awhile. If the need arises, they do make two 20-pound cuffs, which are also widely available.

As far as cost, I have priced these cuffs at a lot of places and the average cost is around twenty dollars for a pair – not a bad investment considering one pair should last for years with normal use.

How much weight should I start off with?

For reasons we've discussed earlier in this chapter, I recommend you shoot for doing one set of an exercise for ten to twenty repetitions. Therefore, you should start out with a weight that allows you to do a minimum of ten repetitions, but no more than twenty. But how do you figure that out?

Well, by a little trial and error. The first time you do a particular exercise, you're just going to have to take your best guess at to how much weight will allow you to do between 10 and 20 repetitions, try the exercise, and then see how it goes. As an example, say you're going to try one of the quadriceps exercises and decide to try two pounds, begin lifting it, and find you can do 15 repetitions in good form. That's great – you've hit our target range of 10 to 20 reps! Next time, you'll then use two pounds again, and try to do a few more reps, eventually working up to 20 reps before adding more weight.

The other thing that commonly happens when you're doing an exercise for the first time, is that you might find it's either too heavy (maybe you could lift it only once or twice) *or* it's way too light (maybe you could lift it twenty-five times or more). Here again, that's not a big problem. When trying the exercise the next time, simply take another good guess, and then adjust the weight up or down a little as needed. Do keep in mind that when *anyone* starts a weight-training program, or tries a new exercise for the first time, it's perfectly normal for it to take one or two exercise sessions to find the appropriate weight.

Like I said, it'll be a matter of a little trial and error at first, but do keep in mind that when it comes to strengthening your quadriceps, the main idea is not to see how much weight you can lift, but rather to find a safe starting weight, and then *gradually progress* over time.

A Quick Note on *Isometric* Exercise

The guidelines you've just read about apply to those type of strengthening exercises where your muscles contract while you're lifting a weight up and down. In exercise science, this type of exercise is known as *isotonic* exercise.

However what does one do if they need to strengthen their quadriceps, *but they can barely move their knee at all?* Well if this is you, then rest easy. There is yet another proven way to strengthen the quadriceps that involves very little knee motion. Impossible you say? Not really. It's called *isometric* exercise.

The word *isometric* comes from the two Greek words *isos*, meaning "equal" or "like," and *metron*, meaning measure. An isometric exercise, then, is one in which the length of the muscle stays the same as it is contracting. A good example of this is when you use your hand and arm to push hard against a brick wall. Your arm is still and unable to move because you can't push the wall over, yet, there is a definite building up of tension in your muscles that can be used as a type of resistance exercise.

But can something so simple as pushing on an immovable object *really* make one stronger? You bet it can or it wouldn't be in this book. Here are a couple of studies that may surprise a few readers...

- 20 subjects were randomly assigned to either an exercise group or a control group (Carolan 1992)

- those in the exercise group did 30 isometric contractions of their quadriceps muscles per a day, three days a week, for 8 weeks

- the control group did not exercise

- results showed that only those subjects that did the isometric exercise increased the strength of their quadriceps muscle by a whopping 33%

and...

- 15 subjects were randomly assigned to either an exercise group or a control group (Garfinkel 1992)
- those in the exercise group did 30 isometric contractions of their quadriceps muscles per a day, three days a week, for 8-weeks
- the control group did not exercise
- all subjects had CT scans taken of their mid-thigh to see if their muscles had gotten any bigger
- researchers found that after 8-weeks, those subjects who did the isometric exercise had quadriceps muscles that were 15% *bigger* and 28% *stronger*!

With proof that isometrics can *truly* make a person's quadriceps bigger and stronger, it's just the perfect type of strengthening exercise for those readers who have such a painful knee that they can hardly bend or move it around at all.

So what exactly does isometric exercise involve anyway? Well, not much. The exercise in this book merely requires a person to put their knee in a specific position, and then push down against a rolled-up pillow. Pretty easy, huh?

Now as far as how long and how many times you push, as well as how often, we'll once again be using evidence-based guidelines taken straight from multiple randomized controlled trials which have proven that isometrics can indeed increase muscle size and strength. They are:

- push as hard as you comfortably can for 3-5 seconds
- repeat for a total of 30 times, once a day
- do this three times a week

And with this last bit of strength-training information, we're all finished covering the basics. So, now that we're all on the same page, let's move on to some of the best quadriceps strengthening exercises medical research has to offer...

Quadriceps Strengthening Exercise: Option 1
~Isometric on Pillow~

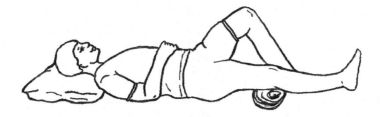

✓ get into the position as the above picture. You can either recline on your elbows or lie flat on your back.

✓ fold a pillow in half, and place it under the knee of the leg that is straight, as shown. If this doesn't feel right, you can do the exercise without the pillow, with your knee straight.

✓ press down as hard as you comfortably can into the pillow with the knee that is straight, and hold for 3-5 seconds. The muscle on the top of your leg, above the kneecap (the quadriceps), should tighten up.

✓ do this 30 times in a row, once a day

✓ repeat the exercise three times a week, separated by a day of rest in between sessions (either Monday-Wednesday-Friday or Tuesday-Thursday-Saturday)

✓ if necessary, work up to the 30 repetitions by adding a few more reps each session until your reach 30

Quadriceps Strengthening Exercise: Option 2
~ Chair Leg Extension~

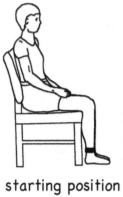 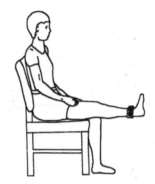 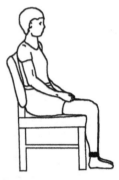

starting position   finishing position

✓ sit in a stationary chair with your back supported as in the starting position

✓ holding on to the chair as needed, kick your leg out as straight as is comfortably possible like the middle picture – *but do not lock it out completely.* Hold for 1-2 seconds, and then slowly lower your leg to the floor. Repeat, working up to twenty times in a row, once a day.

✓ if you can only kick your leg out just a little, that's okay. In time, as any pain you have lessens, and you become stronger and more flexible, you will be able to kick it out farther.

✓ do this exercise three times a week, separated by a day of rest in between sessions (either Monday-Wednesday-Friday or Tuesday-Thursday-Saturday)

✓ start out with no weight, and when you can do 20 reps in good form, add a pound or two with your ankle weights to challenge the quadriceps muscle to get stronger

Quadriceps Strengthening Exercise: Option 3
~ Leg Extension Machine~

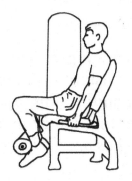 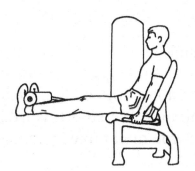 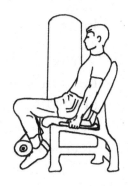

starting position   finishing position

Readers who have access to a gym that has weight machines can substitute the chair leg extension exercise on the last page for the *leg extension machine*. This is because the knee motion is the same, and so it still works the quadriceps muscle. While leg extension machines can vary a bit from place to place, they all look similar to the one in the above picture.

Since it is important that the leg extension machine's seat be adjusted appropriately to each individual, it is suggested that the reader consult with knowledgeable staff at their gym facility to help them set the seat and learn how to use the machine correctly. Know that if you do choose to use the leg extension machine instead of the chair leg extension exercise, the same exercise guidelines still apply...

- ✓ work up to 20 repetitions. When you can do 20 reps in good form, add some weight.

- ✓ do only one set, one time a day

- ✓ do the leg extension machine three times a week, separated by a day of rest in between sessions (either Monday-Wednesday-Friday or Tuesday-Thursday-Saturday)

And there you have it, three exercises that can strengthen your quadriceps muscles. All you need to do now is pick the one that works best for you (depending on your preference, what agrees with your knee, and what equipment you have available) – and then begin!

Noticeable strength gains start after several weeks, with bigger gains becoming apparent after about six to eight weeks of consistent training according to studies. By doing one of these exercises and "tuning up" your quads, you'll be taking a big step towards preventing injury and decreasing any knee pain you might have – *the research has proven it!*

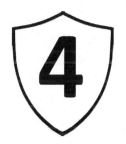

STEP TWO: FINE-TUNE CONTROL OVER YOUR KNEE

Having strong quads is *crucial* in order to have a bulletproof knee. Piles of research support quadriceps strengthening to better a knee, and if I had to pick *just one* knee muscle to strengthen to improve a knee, the quadriceps muscle would be it. Interestingly enough, however, emerging knee research is now showing us that there just might be a few more muscles that would be worth our while to tune-up in order to get a bulletproof knee – muscles that aren't *anywhere* around your knee. In fact, they're actually a little farther north, at your *hip*, and when they're weak, they could cause problems...

- a group of runners with patellofemoral pain syndrome were compared to a group of people with pain-free knees (Ferber 2011)

- researchers tested the strength of all the subject's hip muscles. Markers were also attached to subject's legs at various spots – so the researchers could then conduct a computer analysis of how everybody's knees moved as they ran on a treadmill.

- results showed that the group with patellofemoral pain syndrome had hip muscles that were much weaker than the group with no pain. Calculations also showed that there was much variation in how their knee joints moved from step-to-step.

- interestingly, after strengthening certain hip muscles for only 3 weeks, the group with patellofemoral pain syndrome had a 43% *reduction* in pain **and re-testing showed that their knee motion was much more consistent (less variation) from step-to-step.**

That's interesting. Here you have a group of people with knee pain, weak hip muscles, and knees that don't move the same way from step to step. Then, you strengthen certain hip muscles, and not only does the pain decrease, but their knees start moving less erratically and in a much more consistent pattern!

If you're impressed that stronger hip muscles can control the knee better, you're also going to like this...

- this time, fifteen healthy subjects had the strength of their hip muscles tested. Markers were attached to their legs at various spots, and seven high-speed cameras filmed their knees as they ran (Snyder 2009).

- after this testing, subjects completed a 6-week hip muscle strengthening program – after which time they were tested *again*.

- results showed that hip muscle strength increased after the 6-week program, ***and calculations showed that there was decreased loading on the knee joint as they ran.***

So here again we have another great effect on the knee when we strengthen certain hip muscles – less force on the knee joint! According to these studies, it seems to break down like this...

strengthen the hip muscles

↓

gets you better control of knee motion

↓

results in more consistent knee movements

↓

decreased forces on the knee joint

And if that still isn't enough reason for us to sit up and take notice of the hip muscles in our quest to bulletproof our knees, yet other research has shown that strengthening them can be another valuable tool when it comes to fighting painful knees...

- one study showed that when 24 distance runners with iliotibial band syndrome (a common cause of pain on the side of the knee) completed a 6-week rehabilitation program with special attention to hip muscle strengthening, *22 of the 24 athletes became pain-free* (Fredericson 2000)

- in another study, 40 individuals with painful knee arthritis reported *decreased knee pain after finishing an 8-week hip strengthening program* (Sled 2010)

- when 14 females with patellofemoral pain syndrome completed an 8-week hip strengthening program, they found that their pain significantly decreased, *and remained significantly decreased 6 months later* (Khayambashi 2012)

As a researcher, I'd like to see more studies done in the future to solidify the use of hip muscle strengthening in the treatment of knee pain, like we have for the quads, but for now, we do have some very good biomechanical and clinical studies showing us its well-worth our time to invest in a hip strengthening exercise to bulletproof our knees.

Now as you might have noticed, I have been saying "hip muscle strengthening" thus far in this chapter. But which hip muscles do we specifically need to worry about? All of them, or just a few?

Well, there's one hip muscle in particular that keeps coming up again and again in all the studies we've been talking about. It's called a *hip abductor.* Sound weird? Let's start at the beginning...

Hip Abduction

Abduction is a motion – more specifically, it's when you're moving a body part *away* from your midline. Hip abduction, then, is when you're moving your leg away from your body, out to the side. A picture is worth a thousand words, soooo...

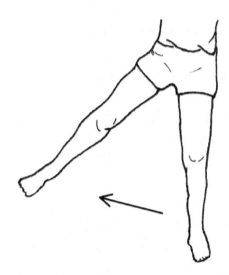

Figure 20. This person is *abducting* their right leg.

And it makes no difference if you're standing or lying, if you're moving your leg out to the side, well, it's still hip abduction...

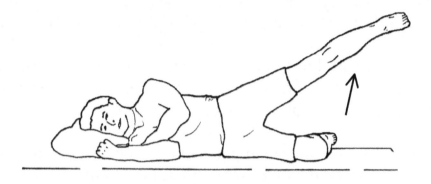

Figure 21. This person is *abducting* their left leg.

So now you know what hip abduction is. The next thing you need to know is that there's a little muscle in your hip that is key in helping you perform this motion. It's known as the *gluteus medius* – and it's the hip muscle we're most concerned about strengthening. Here's a picture of where it's at and what it looks like...

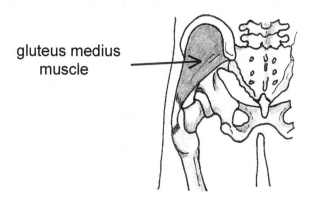

gluteus medius muscle

Figure 22. Looking at the right hip from the front – the gluteus medius muscle.

While the gluteus medius is a relatively small muscle, it can cause some *big* problems if it's weak. Because it attaches to your pelvis as well as your leg bone, it also has the job of keeping your hips and pelvis level as you walk.

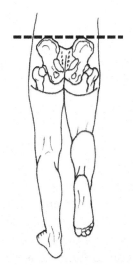

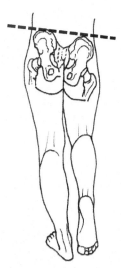

Figure 23. A strong gluteus medius helps to keep the pelvis level as you walk or run

Figure 24. A weak gluteus medius can cause the pelvis to tilt as you walk. In this case, the right hip drops because the *left* gluteus medius is weak and can't hold it up.

The point to all this is not to give you a biomechanics lesson, but rather to let you know how weakness in a muscle *way up* at the hip can cause alignment problems – and influence the rest of your leg.

Having said that, it's time now for me to show you how to strengthen your gluteus medius. Without further delay, here's the *sidelying hip abduction exercise* that comes directly from the studies you've just been reading about...

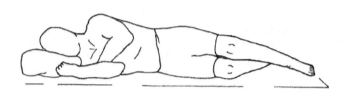

- Find a comfortable place to lay down (the floor or on a bed will do).
- Get into the position in the picture.
- The person in the picture is about to exercise the *left* gluteus medius.

- Now, keeping your knee straight, raise your leg up slowly. It should take you 3-4 seconds to raise your leg up.
- You don't need to go any higher than the picture shows.

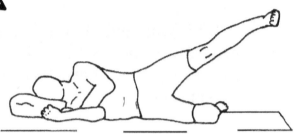

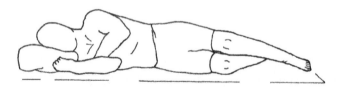

- Return your leg to the starting position – you've just done one repetition.
- Repeat, working up to 20 times in a row.
- When you can do this 20 times in a row, in good form, add a 1 or 2 pound ankle weight to challenge the muscle to get stronger.
- As you continue to add more weight over time, your gluteus medius will become stronger and stronger.
- Do the exercise 1 time a day, 3 times a week, with a day of rest in between – for example Monday, Wednesday, Friday, or Tuesday, Thursday, Saturday

For those readers who have access to a gym, they do make machines that can strengthen your gluteus medius – simply because you're still abducting your leg when using it. While you will find slight variations between models, a *hip abduction machine* will look very similar to the one below…

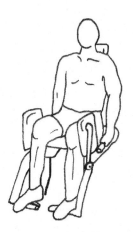

- Get into the position in the picture.
- Set the machine on the lowest amount of weight to start out with.
- You will be working *both* gluteus medius muscles at the same time.
- Notice that the pads you push against with your knees should be on the *outside* of the knee, not the inside.

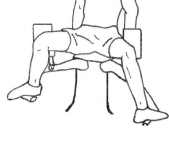

- Now, push *outward* against the pads with both knees at the same time, as far as you can comfortably. It should take you 3-4 seconds to do this.
- You don't need to spread your legs apart any farther than the picture shows.

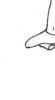

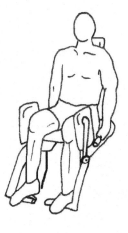

- Return your leg to the starting position – you've just done one repetition.
- Repeat, working up to 20 times in a row.
- When you can do this 20 times in a row, add 1 or 2 pounds to the machine to make the muscle stronger.
- As you continue to add more weight over time, your gluteus medius will become stronger and stronger.
- Do the exercise 1 time a day, 3 times a week with a day of rest in between – for example Monday, Wednesday, Friday, or Tuesday, Thursday, Saturday.

By doing a targeted hip exercise and using the evidence-based strength guidelines in this chapter, you'll be fine tuning control over your knee joint - and one step closer to a bulletproof knee!

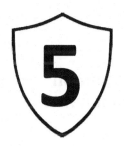

STEP THREE: OPTIMIZE KNEE FLEXIBILTIY

So far we've talked about bulletproofing your knee by strengthening specific muscles. However, if you stopped there and just did those two exercises, you would *not* have a bulletproof knee. Why? Because the strongest, most stable knee in the world is practically useless if all it can do is move around a few degrees in each direction. While most of us can probably move our knees around fairly well, a bulletproof knee is one that has *optimal* flexibility in *all* the major directions.

Why Your Knee Might Not Be As Flexible As It Should Be

Every reader will most likely have a slightly different amount of tightness in his or her knee. Some might not be able to stretch their knee out fully, while others may have difficulty bending it back very far. The specific stretches in this chapter will help you restore all the major motions in your knee, getting it up to peak performance. But first, what kinds of things would prevent a knee from moving freely in all directions?

Well, there are lots of reasons why people can lack flexibility in their knees, and no two readers may have the exact same cause. On the next page is a table that lists some common reasons why knee motion can be limited...

Problems that may lead to a loss of knee flexibility	Possible causes of this problem	Common Treatments
Swelling	Fluid in the knee joint that takes up space and prevents full motion.	Ice, stretching, removal of fluid by needle, anti-inflammatory medications
Tight Muscles	Muscles become shorter when not regularly stretched through their full range of motion.	Stretching exercises
Mechanical Problems	Problems such as torn cartilage or loose bodies in the joint can block normal motion between the bones.	In some situations, surgical removal
Pain	A knee that hurts doesn't move through a full range of motion, causing muscles and other structures to shorten over time.	Exercise, pain medications
Tight Joint Capsule	The tissue that surrounds the entire joint can become tight, keeping the bones from moving normally.	Stretching, joint manipulation

You can see from the list that there are various causes of lost knee motion – and, likewise, various treatments to correct these problems. Although this is a do-it-yourself book, I would like to make it clear that not all cases can be treated conservatively at home. For instance, a person who has a loose body, such as a piece of torn cartilage in his or her knee – a problem that can mechanically block knee motion much like a marble in a gearbox – could quite possibly need surgery. Realistically, though, most people with this type of problem will probably not be reading this book, but rather end up at the doctor's office, because it will be obvious that something major has gone wrong. Indeed, many readers with decreased knee motion can be more than adequately treated with a simple stretching program, done correctly. My only point here is to let you know that although stretching is indicated most frequently in the vast majority of cases, it is not a universal treatment. Please consult your medical professional should any questions arise.

Some readers may also have noticed that what is missing from the list of causes are specific ailments such as arthritis. That is because in this book we're more concerned with function rather than labels. Therefore, when looking at why a knee isn't able to be bent backward fully, we don't say it's because of arthritis, but rather because of the pain, swelling, or muscle tightness that's secondary to arthritis. And why is it a good idea to think about it like this? Because doing so helps us better zero in on specific *functional* problems we can treat.

The Three Motions of Your Knee

Okay. Now that you know what can limit knee flexibility, we need to talk about which knee motions need to be improved the most. So how many different ways does your knee move anyway?

Well, while most people think of your knee as only being able to swing back and forth like a door hinge, the truth is that your knee actually *rotates* as well. Although this may seem a bit unbelievable, the truth is that with each step you take, your lower leg bone (the tibia) actually rotates *outward*. On the next page is a neat little test you can do that demonstrates this little-known knee motion...

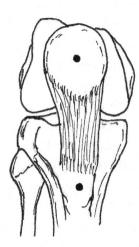

Figure 25. What the right knee looks like from the front when your knee is *bent*. Note that the dots are in line with each other

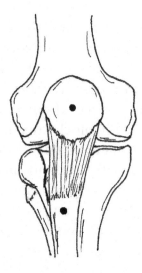

Figure 26. What the right knee looks like from the front when your knee is *straight*. Note that the lower dot has moved to the side.

The Helfet Test

- to try the above test, sit down *with your knee bent at a right angle.* Then, take a pen and put a dot in the middle of your kneecap (top dot).

- next, put another mark on the bony bump that sticks out on the lower leg just below your kneecap (lower dot)

- make sure the dots are in line with each other as in Figure 25

- now, while still sitting, kick your leg out

- your knee should now be straight and the dots should look like Figure 26

- note that the dots are no longer in a straight line. This is because your lower leg bone has rotated *outward* as you straightened your leg. This same motion also occurs as you are walking.

Pretty nifty test, huh? I discovered that one years ago in an old book I came across while I was digging around in the medical library. Now if you did find that your knee was too tight to do the test, don't worry, the stretching exercises in this chapter can most certainly help you regain normal flexibility.

Okay, so that's *one* of the three major knee motions. The last two are *extension*, which is the motion of straightening out your knee...

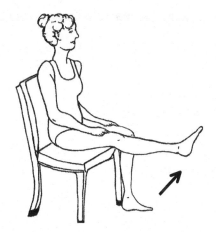

Figure 27. A person with their right knee in extension. The motion of extension is when one is *straightening* their knee.

and *flexion*, which is when you're bending your knee...

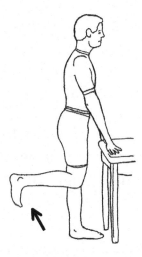

Figure 28. A person with their right knee in flexion. The motion of flexion is when one is *bending* their knee.

How Much Motion Should a
Normal Knee Have Anyway?

The range of motion a normal knee is supposed to have depends very much on which source you happen to be consulting at the moment. Take a look at the following list I compiled one time from several different publications and you'll see what I mean...

Source	Normal amount of knee bending
American Academy of Orthopaedic Surgeons (1965)	135°
Clark (1920)	145°
Daniels and Worthingham (1972)	130°
Journal of the American Medical Association (1958)	120°
Kapandji (1970)	160°
Kendall and McCreary (1983)	140°

As with many questions, the answer seems to depend upon whom you talk to. If pushed in a corner, I'd have to say that the most commonly quoted number from most of the literature I've looked at is 135 degrees. This means that most people should be able to pull their heel back towards their rear end to an angle of 135 degrees. As for extension, the motion of straightening the leg, few would disagree that a normal knee should be able to at least be able to straighten the leg out all the way, making a perfectly straight line.

With all the apparent confusion over what's considered "normal," there is another way of approaching the whole issue. Rather than trying to increase our knee flexibility to a controversial "normal" range, maybe we should be more concerned about how much knee motion we actually need for our day-to-day activities - and just shoot for this as our personal standard.

Looking into this very matter, Dr. Phillip Rowe, of the Queen Margaret University College, and his colleagues conducted a very insightful study that determined exactly how much knee flexibility is necessary for us to be able to normally go about our daily business. Hooking up the knees of twenty healthy individuals to a fancy device called a *flexible goniometer*, these researchers followed subjects around and recorded their knee motion as they performed eleven common activities. When all was said and done, here's what the study found...

Activity	Maximum amount of knee bending needed on average
walking of level ground	67°
walking up a 5° slope	65°
walking down a 5° slope	72°
climbing a 20-step flight of stairs	99°
going down a 20-step flight of stairs	97°
sitting down in a regular (18¼ inch high) chair	99°
getting up from a regular chair	99°
sitting down into a low chair (about 15 inches high)	102°
getting up from a low chair	105°
getting into a bathtub	131°

Readers with substantial losses of flexibility can use the above information to determine roughly how much range of motion they'll need in their knees for a particular activity, and this information will indicate how much flexibility they'll need to aim for with the stretching exercises. For instance, if you are having difficulty climbing stairs, the table tells us that your knees, on average, must be able to bend about 99 degrees to adequately perform that activity. To walk on level ground, your minimum goal would be about 67 degrees, and so on. Keep in mind that these are for *normal* daily activities. A reader who needs to function at a high level, such as an athlete – a hurdler, for example – probably needs the highest degree of knee motion that she or he can get.

When estimating how flexible your own knee is, use the 0-degree and 90-degree marks as points of reference. Zero degrees is a knee that is extended perfectly straight, while a knee bending at 90 degrees makes a right angle, or "L" shape. From here, you can roughly estimate other points, such as 45-degrees (halfway between 0 and 90 degrees) or 135 degrees (halfway between 90 degrees and the back of the thigh).

Stretching Secrets That Work

While there are many different techniques to choose from when it comes to stretching out a tight muscle and improving knee motions, by far the easiest and least complicated way is known as *the static stretch*. A static (or stationary) stretch takes a tight muscle, puts it in a lengthened position, and keeps it there for a certain period of time. For instance, if you wanted to use the static stretch technique to make your back muscles more flexible, you could simply lie on your back and pull your knees to your chest. Thus, as you are holding this position, the back muscles are being *statically stretched*. There's no bouncing, just a gentle, sustained stretch.

It sounds easy, perhaps a bit *too* easy, so you may be wondering at this point just how effective static stretching really is when it comes to making one more flexible?

Well, a quick review of the stretching research pretty much lays it out straight as there are *multiple* randomized controlled trials clearly in agreement that this is a winning method. Here are the highlights...

- a study published in the journal *Physical Therapy* took 57 subjects and randomly divided them up into four groups (Bandy 1994)

- the first group held their static stretch for a length of 15 seconds, the second group for 30 seconds, and the third for 60. The fourth group (the control group) did not stretch at all.

- all three groups performed *one* stretch a day, five days a week, for six weeks

- results showed that holding a stretch for a period of 30 seconds was just as effective at increasing flexibility as holding one for 60 seconds. Also, holding a stretch for a period of 30 seconds was much more effective than holding one for 15 seconds or (of course) not stretching at all.

Hmm. Looks like if you hold a stretch for 15 seconds, it doesn't do much to make you more flexible. On the other hand, holding a stretch for 30 full seconds *does* work – and just as well as 60 seconds!

Wow. So now that we know that 30 seconds seems to be the magic number, makes you wonder if doing *a bunch* of 30-second stretches would be *even better* than doing it one time a day like they did in the study...

- another randomized controlled trial done several years later (Bandy 1997) set out to research not only the optimal length of time to hold a static stretch, *but also the optimal number of times to do it*
- 93 subjects were recruited and randomly placed into one of five groups: 1) perform three 1-minute stretches; 2) perform three 30-second stretches; 3) perform a 1-minute stretch; 4) perform a 30-second stretch; or 5) do no stretching at all (the control group)
- the results? Not so surprising was the fact that all groups that stretched became more flexible than the control group that didn't stretch.
- however what *was* surprising was the finding that among the groups that did stretch, no one group became more flexible than the other!
- in other words, the researchers found that as far as trying to become more flexible, it made no difference whether the stretching time was increased from 30 to 60 seconds, OR when the frequency was changed from doing one stretch a day to doing three stretches a day

So here we have yet *another* randomized controlled trial (the kind of study that provides the highest form of proof in medicine) which is showing us *once again* that holding a stretch for 30 seconds is *just as effective* as holding it for 60 seconds. And to top it all off, doing the 30-second stretch *once* a day is just as good as if you did it three times!

Other randomized controlled trials have also supported the amazing effectiveness of the 30-second stretch done one time a day, five days a week, to make one more flexible (Bandy 1998), and interestingly enough, a more recent study showed that doing one 30-second stretch once a day, ***three times a week*** can even make you a little more flexible (Davis 2005) – good to know if you're having a busy week and happen to miss a day or two of stretching!

So as the randomized controlled trials *clearly* point out, it really doesn't take a lot of time to stretch out tight muscles *if* you know how. Based on the current published stretching research, this book recommends the following guidelines for the average person needing to stretch out a tight muscle with the *static stretch technique*:

* **get into the starting position**
* **next, begin moving into the stretch position until a *gentle* stretch is felt**
* **once this position is achieved, hold for a full 30 seconds**
* **when the 30 seconds is up, *slowly* release the stretch**
* **do this one time a day, five days a week**

One last note. While it is acceptable to feel a little discomfort while doing a stretch, it is *not* okay to be in pain. Do not force yourself to get into any stretching position, and by all means, skip the stretch entirely if it makes any pain worse.

It Only Takes Two Stretches To Get the Job Done

Okay, time for the meat and potatoes of the chapter – the stretching exercises! There are two main muscle groups that we're most concerned about when it comes to restoring knee flexibility – the hamstrings and the quadriceps...

* *the quadriceps muscles.* Put your hand on the front of your thigh and you'll be right on them. If they're tight, they can keep you from being able to bend your leg back to your buttocks. Therefore, stretching them will improve your knee *flexion.*

- *the hamstrings muscles.* If you put your hand on the back of your thigh, you're right on these muscles. If they're tight, they can keep your leg from straightening your leg out all the way. Therefore, stretching them out will improve your knee *extension*.

To take into account the diverse abilities of different readers (some may have difficulty standing up to do a stretch, while others may have trouble lying on their back), I have provided illustrations of how to stretch the hamstrings and quadriceps muscles in *several* different positions. Pick the stretch that is done in the position that is easiest for you – and know that they're all equally effective, provided you use the evidence-based stretching guidelines we covered earlier in the chapter. On the next few pages are the stretches with detailed guidelines for doing each one...

Quadriceps Stretch #1

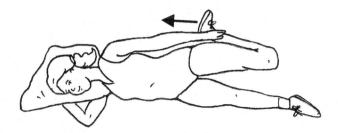

1. Get into the same position as the above picture. It's okay to be on a bed or on the floor.

2. Grab your ankle and pull your foot backward toward your buttocks until you feel a gentle stretch in the *front* of your thigh.

3. You can bring your knee backward for an even stronger stretch.

4. Hold for 30 full seconds.

5. Do this once a day, five days a week. It's okay to work up to the 30 seconds if you have to.

Quadriceps Stretch #2

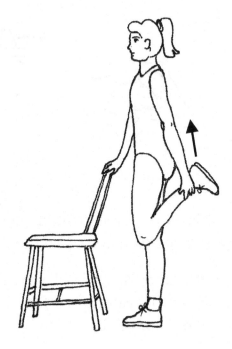

1. Get into the same position as the above picture. Use a sturdy chair or perhaps a countertop.

2. Grab your ankle and pull your foot backward toward your buttocks until you feel a gentle stretch in the *front* of your thigh.

3. You can bring your knee backward for an even stronger stretch.

4. Hold for 30 full seconds.

5. Do this once a day, five days a week. It's okay to work up to the 30 seconds if you have to.

Hamstring Stretch #1

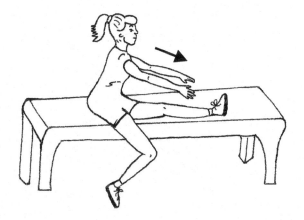

1. Get into the same position as the above picture. It's okay to be on a bed or on the floor.

2. Keeping your back straight, lean forward toward your foot until you feel a gentle stretch on the *back* of your thigh. Try to bend forward from the hips as much as possible, rather than bending from your low back.

3. Try to keep your knee straight.

4. Hold for 30 full seconds.

5. Do this once a day, five days a week. It's okay to work up to the 30 seconds if you have to.

Hamstring Stretch #2

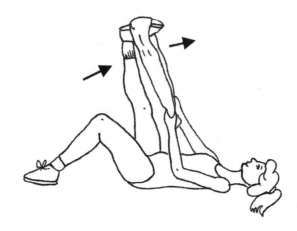

1. Using a towel, get into the above position. It's okay to be on a bed or on the floor.

2. Pull your foot toward you until you feel a gentle stretch in the *back* of your thigh.

3. Try to keep your knee straight.

4. Hold for 30 full seconds.

5. Do this once a day, five days a week. It's okay to work up to the 30 seconds if you have to.

By stretching, you will be sending a clear signal to your muscles that they need to elongate. Then, over a period of weeks, the tissues will begin to gradually lengthen bit-by-bit.

Pretty simple, huh? If you use the guidelines provided, stretching to lengthen the muscles that provide mobility to your knee doesn't have to be an all-day affair. Also, remember to pick only one stretch for your hamstrings muscle group, and one stretch for your quadriceps. Therefore, you should be doing a grand total of only two stretches a day, taking you sixty seconds to complete (thirty seconds per exercise) – a minimal investment of your time in an activity that is going to give you a much more efficient working knee!

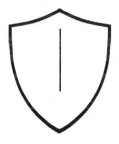

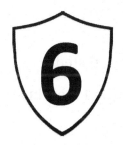

STEP FOUR: INCREASE *DYNAMIC* KNEE STABILITY

Having good *dynamic knee stability* means that you can keep your knee stable as you are moving it around and putting it into action. No matter if you're running on uneven ground, suddenly walking on a slippery floor, or climbing stairs, well, your knee is just able to react quickly – and contract the right muscles in order to keep it in a safe and stable position. And it's essential in order to have a bulletproof knee.

But contrary to popular belief, dynamic knee stability isn't just a matter of pure strength. In other words, having very strong leg muscles isn't enough – it involves *other* factors. A good example of this comes from people who have ruptured their ACL, or anterior cruciate ligament.

Recall from the first chapter that more than half of those who rupture this ligament can be classified as a *non-coper,* that is they have significant knee instability, even during daily activities, and complain of the knee frequently giving way.

On the other hand, there are those known as *copers,* who have also ruptured their ACL, but can still maintain high levels of activity. The knee does not give-way, even while doing things such as jumping or pivoting. Furthermore, these lucky individuals are able to return to pre-injury activities *without* surgery.

So here we have two groups of people who have identical ACL tears, yet one group has *poor* dynamic knee stability (the non-copers), and the other has *good* dynamic knee stability (the copers). Now it's been the topic of much research – the differences between the copers and non-copers – and we have found some pretty interesting things...

- in one study, researchers compared 11 copers to 10 non-copers to 10 healthy people (Rudolph 2001)

- the strength of subject's quadriceps muscles were tested

- as subjects walked and jogged, six cameras recorded their knee motions so they could be analyzed

- muscle activation patterns were also assessed with surface electrodes which were attached to the leg muscles – these recorded the electrical activity of the muscles as subjects walked and jogged. Therefore, it could be determined what muscles were contracting when.

Sounds like a pretty thorough study, doesn't it? Well, when the study was completed, the researchers found several important differences between the copers and the non-copers....

- *the non-copers had weaker quadriceps than the copers.* This should be no surprise after reading Chapter 3 – weak quads are usually associated with decreased function and pain, while strong quads usually mean improved function and less pain.

- *the non-copers moved their knees much differently than the copers, and activated their knee muscles in a different pattern.* Interestingly, the non-copers used a "knee stiffening strategy" to try and stabilize their injured knees. Copers, on the other hand, moved like uninjured people with normal knee motions.

At this point, some readers might be thinking that since the non-copers had weaker leg muscles (the quads), maybe that's why they were moving their knees so much differently than the copers? And so all we have to do is just strengthen the quads to fix the stability problem?

A good thought, and certainly quad strengthening is a must. But it turns out that if you add something else, something called *perturbation training* to the mix, things turn out *even better...*

- 26 patients who had either a ruptured ACL, or ruptured ACL graft (a graft is a tissue that has surgically replaced a torn ACL ligament) were included in this study (Fitzgerald 2000)

- 14 subjects were randomized to a standard rehabilitation program, which included strengthening exercises for the quads

- the other 12 subjects were randomized to also complete the standard program *plus perturbation training*

- at the end of the study, only 50% of those who completed the standard program were able to return to full activity, and did not report an episode of their knee giving way

- on the other hand, *92% of those who completed the standard program **plus perturbation training** returned to full activity, and did not report an episode of their knee giving way*

What a difference in success rates – *92% versus 50%* - when you add perturbation training! Talk about increasing dynamic knee stability in some of the most unstable knees a physical therapist can see – those with torn ligaments. And it gets even better...

- another study compared 17 people with *complete* ACL ruptures to 17 healthy controls (Chmielewski 2005)

- six cameras recorded the knee motions of all subjects as they walked so movement patterns could be analyzed

- muscle activation patterns were also assessed with surface electrodes which were attached to the leg muscles – these recorded electrical activity of the muscles as subjects walked

- both groups underwent a program of perturbation training

- data showed that before perturbation training, those with torn ACL's used a knee stiffening strategy to try and stabilize their knees as they walked (a stiff knee equals less motion)

- however, *after* perturbation training, *those with torn ACL's moved with much less knee stiffness, and their walking patterns more closely resembled those of the healthy controls subjects*

From these studies, all published in peer-reviewed journals, it's obvious that perturbation training can without a doubt improve dynamic knee stability in people with some of the worst knee problems – which makes it a tool we can definitely use to help bulletproof our knees. So what exactly does perturbation training involve anyway?

In a nutshell, perturbation exercises put your knee in a stable position while you are standing, and then you try to keep it there as an outside force "perturbs" (or disturbs) your balance. Thus, by trying to maintain a stable knee position as controlled forces are trying to "throw off your balance", everything that goes into knee stability is challenged – such as the coordination of muscle contractions. Just as lifting a weight challenges a muscle to get stronger, challenging your knee with controlled "perturbations" increases its dynamic stability.

The other thing that perturbation training also does, is improve your *proprioception*. Pronounced pro-pree-o-ception, all this fourteen-letter word means is the ability you have at any given moment to sense the position and movements of your body. For example, if you close your eyes, you could probably tell me without much difficulty if your elbow is bent or straight, or if your head is turned to the left or right – all without even looking.

To give you more of an idea of just how critical proprioception is, here are a few everyday activities whose success or failure depends on the proper functioning of your sense of *proprioception*...

- getting something out of your pocket
- pushing down on the gas or brake pedal in your car
- walking in the dark
- scratching that hard-to-reach spot on your back

As you can see, all of these activities involve doing something without the help of your vision. By giving your brain constant updates as to the position of your body parts, your proprioception helps you out a lot when you are unable to see exactly what you are doing.

Another good example of how crucial the sense of proprioception is to our day-to-day lives comes from a patient I had once who lacked proprioception in both of his legs. Unfortunately, this gentleman had a condition known as *CIPD* or *chronic inflammatory demyelinating polyneuropathy*, a rare neurological disorder involving destruction of the covering around the nerves. As his physical therapist, it was my job to get him out of bed and see how well he could walk.

The first hurdle we had to cross, getting him onto his feet, proved to be somewhat easy; we used a walker and his legs were quite strong. Walking, however, turned out to be another matter entirely. Each step was a journey into the unknown. Since his legs gave him little feedback as to where they actually were, his whole leg would begin to swing wildly in a circular motion as he desperately tried to place his foot on the floor. Even though he knew where he wanted his legs to go – and had plenty of strength to make them move, it was impractical for him to walk any meaningful distance without proprioception.

As you can see, there is much we would be unable to do without our sense of proprioception. Your average person with a knee problem, however, will have nowhere near the kind of proprioception problems my patient had. Having proprioception problems to the degree he suffered usually occurs when one has a serious problem with his or her nervous system. Perhaps that is why proprioception exercises are usually either last on the list of treatments for the knee, or are neglected entirely.

While a lot of medical professionals tend to think of proprioception problems as happening only in patients with grave neurological disorders, nothing could be farther from the truth. For instance, a quick look at the knee research shows us that proprioception deficits have been found frequently in people with *many* different kinds of knee problems...

- people with patellofemoral pain syndrome
- people with knee osteoarthritis
- people who have ruptured their ACL
- people who have dislocated their kneecap
- people who have torn their medial meniscus

Apparently knee problems and proprioception problems can go hand-in-hand, and so we have lots of reasons to make sure that our proprioception is up to par when it comes to bulletproofing a knee. But in case you need one more reason, consider this. Say you're merrily walking along with a friend and are temporarily distracted as you're talking. Suddenly, you happen to step off a curb you didn't know was there. This catches you off guard, and sends a sudden "jolt" through your entire leg and knee joint. What happens next depends to a large degree on how well your proprioception works. Consider the following...

- the knee with *normal* proprioception can send information to the brain about your leg's position and movements in a split second. In turn, the leg muscles can react immediately by contracting to maintain your balance and posture, as well as by stabilizing your knee to keep it in a safe position.

- *on the other hand*, the knee with *decreased* proprioception fails to react nearly as fast, and therefore puts your knee at risk of injury

The point here is that proprioception very much serves a *protective* role too. When the nerves in your knee muscles, tendons, and joint capsule immediately send feedback to your brain as to what's going on, you can then keep things under control and avoid injury. So in short, proprioception helps to protect your knee from injury and joint damage. On the next few pages are a series of exercises that can help you improve your proprioception – as well as your dynamic knee stability...

Dynamic Knee Stability Exercise
Phase I

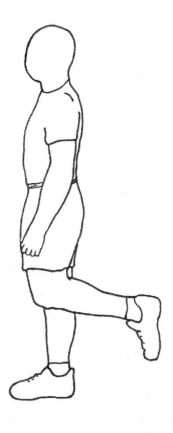

✓ Stand on one leg in the same position as the picture. The knee can be straight or slightly bent, whichever is more comfortable.

✓ If you can't balance well on one leg at all, or if you feel like you might fall, stand next to a table, chair, or doorway – something you can lightly hold on to.

✓ The goal is to *work up* to being able to stand on one leg for 30 full seconds.

✓ Repeat the exercise on the other leg if you wish.

✓ When you can stand on one leg, well-balanced, for 30 full seconds, *without holding on to anything*, it's time to move on to Phase II.

Dynamic Knee Stability Exercise
Phase II

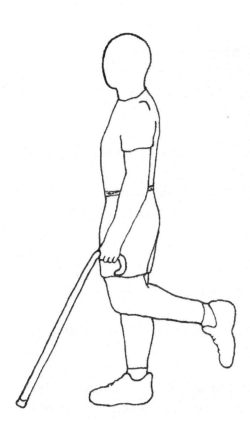

✓ Stand on one leg in the same position as the picture, with a cane in either hand. The knee can be straight or slightly bent, whichever is more comfortable. It's okay for the cane to touch the floor.

✓ Once you are balanced in this position, use the cane to give yourself a gentle push backwards – the idea being to slightly "throw-off" your balance.

✓ Now as this push causes you to slightly lose your balance, try to regain it and get back to the stable starting position in the picture – without using the cane or the other leg that was in the air.

✓ Repeat this over and over, working up to 30 full seconds over time.

✓ The goal is to be able to regain your balance (without using the cane or other leg) while doing a series of these "perturbations" for 30 seconds.

✓ Repeat the exercise on the other leg if you wish.

✓ When you can keep your balance for 30 full seconds of perturbations, move on to phase III.

✓ As you can see, the point of the exercise is to slightly "throw-off" your balance, which in turn challenges the knee you are standing on to try and stabilize itself. You can also experiment with pushing yourself randomly from other directions with the cane, such as from the side or behind you, which really challenges your knee to stabilize itself from forces coming from many different directions.

Dynamic Knee Stability Exercise
Phase III

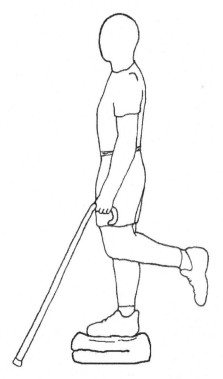

✓ This exercise is done the same way as the one in Phase II, except this time you will make things more challenging by standing on a pillow to make the surface more unstable.

✓ Stand on one leg, on a folded pillow, in the same position as the picture, with a cane in either hand. The knee can be straight or slightly bent, whichever is more comfortable. It's okay for the cane to touch the floor.

✓ Once you are balanced in this position, use the cane to give yourself a gentle push backwards – the idea being to slightly "throw-off" your balance.

✓ Now as this push causes you to slightly lose your balance, try to regain it and get back to the stable starting position in the picture – without using the cane or the other leg that was in the air.

✓ Repeat this over and over, working up to 30 full seconds over time.

✓ The goal is to regain your balance (without using the cane or other leg) while doing a series of these "perturbations" for 30 seconds.

✓ Repeat the exercise on the other leg if you wish.

✓ Once again, the point of the exercise is to slightly "throw-off" your balance, which in turn challenges the knee you are standing on to try and stabilize itself – this time on a slightly unstable surface (the pillow). You can also experiment with pushing yourself randomly from other directions with the cane, such as from the side or behind you, which really challenges your knee to stabilize itself from forces coming from many different directions. For an added challenge, consider increasing the time to a full 60 seconds.

Although these exercises may seem simple, I think most readers will find them more challenging than they look. Since there is little research telling us how often a person needs to do these exercises to get *the best* results, I recommend doing them three times a week with a day of rest in between, just as with the strengthening exercises. Week by week, the exercises will begin to get easier and easier – indicating that you're well on your way to improving your proprioception and dynamic knee stability.

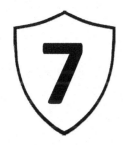

THE BULLETPROOF KNEE PROGRAM

The first chapter of this book explained the idea of the *bulletproof knee* - a knee that is *pain-free* and *resistant to injury*. It put forth the principle that, knee pain is the result of something not functioning properly, and that if the function is restored, pain will go away. Likewise, improving knee function also has the added benefit of making the knee more resistant to injury. Then we addressed the four specific knee functions that need to be optimized. As you'll recall, we called them "the four abilities." They are as follows...

- ✓ **Superior Quad Strength**
- ✓ **Finely-Tuned Control Over the Knee**
- ✓ **Optimal Flexibility**
- ✓ **Enhanced Dynamic Knee Stability**

The rest of the book then provided you with the tools you need in order to restore and optimize these four abilities, as well as the scientific rationale for using them. In this chapter, we will put all this information together and put it into action.

The Master Plan

This section will help you organize all of the exercises from the preceeding chapters into an effective, time-efficient program, **THE BULLETPROOF KNEE PROGRAM**. Let's start with an overview of a recommended schedule for you to follow...

DO THESE EXERCISES ON MONDAY, WEDNESDAY, and FRIDAY

Exercise to Strengthen the Quads (Pick One)

Isometric on Pillow	**Chair Leg Extension**	**Leg Extension Machine**
		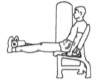
1 set x 30 reps	1 set x 20 reps	1 set x 20 reps

Exercise to Fine-Tune Control Over the Knee (Pick One)

Exercise to Increase Dynamic Knee Stability (Work Through Phases I- II -III)

Hip Abduction Machine   **Sidelying Hip Abduction**

  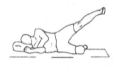   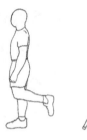

1 set x 20 reps   1 set x 20 reps   1 x day

Exercises to Increase Knee Flexibility (Pick One Stretch for Each Muscle)

Quadriceps Stretch #1	**Quadriceps Stretch #2**	**Hamstrings Stretch #1**	**Hamstrings Stretch #2**
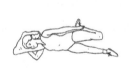	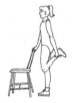	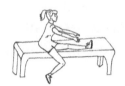	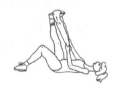
hold for 30 sec. x 1	hold for 30 sec. x 1	hold for 30 sec. x 1	hold for 30 sec. x 1

DO THESE EXERCISES ON TUESDAY and THURSDAY

```
┌─────────────────────────────────────────────┐
│        Exercises to Increase Knee Flexibility │
│         (Pick One Stretch for Each Muscle)    │
└─────────────────────────────────────────────┘
```

Quadriceps Stretch #1	Quadriceps Stretch #2	Hamstrings Stretch #1	Hamstrings Stretch #2
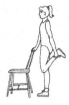	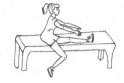		
hold for 30 sec. x 1	hold for 30 sec. x 1	hold for 30 sec. x 1	hold for 30 sec. x 1

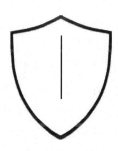

Getting Started

So how exactly do you go about getting started on this plan to bulletproof your knee? Here area a few suggestions...

- First get an okay from your doctor to make sure that the exercises are safe for you to do.

- Next, take a look at the weekly exercise schedule on pages 88 and 89 (the two previous pages).

- Pick a day of the week on which to start.

- Once you've decided when you'll begin, review the detailed breakdown of exercises for that particular day to learn what exercises to do. If you need more detail on how to do any of them, review Chapters 3 through 6 for more extensive instructions.

- On the day you've chosen, jump right in and take the first step toward getting a bulletproof knee!

What to Expect

When I give an exercise program to a patient, they usually want to know how long it will take before they start seeing results. The answer lies in how long it takes the body to adapt to the type of exercises I have given.   In this book, there are three main types of exercises: strengthening exercises, stretching exercises, and stability exercises. As such, there are many published studies showing that your average person can see measurable increases in each of these areas (strength, flexibility, and stability) *in a 6-week time frame*.   Therefore, I would encourage every reader to do THE BULLETPROOF KNEE PROGRAM for at least a full 6-weeks to see highly significant gains of strength, flexibility, and stability in your knee area – as well as a decrease in any knee pain you might be experiencing.

Now if you've seen good progress in 6-weeks' time, but you're still not quite where you want to be, continue with the program until you reach your goal. As long as you continue to do the stretches using a thirty-second hold, and increase the weight when you can do 20 reps in good form, you should see progress.

On the other hand, if your knee is feeling and working great after six-weeks, try doing the strengthening, stretching, and stability exercises one time a week for maintenance, and see how that goes. Make sure that you are using the same weight you've worked up to for once-a-week maintenance, and continue holding the stretches for thirty seconds.

A Final Note

The first exercise program I ever wrote for publication was in my book, *The Multifidus Back Pain Solution*. It consisted of three exercises, and I asked the reader to choose only *one*. The exercises were shown to be effective in randomized controlled trials, and if the diligent reader truly followed my specific, evidence-based guidelines, I could all but guarantee that their back pain would improve, if not go away altogether.

Eventually the book was translated into other languages, and as its popularity grew, I started getting some interesting feedback from worldwide readers. Two points consistently came up regarding the exercise routine:

- there weren't enough exercises in the book
- some of the exercises were too simple, or they were ones that readers had already seen/done before

In case some of these same issues bother you as you reviewed the exercise routine in this chapter, I would like to take a moment out to dispel a few common misconceptions before you get started. The first one is that some people think you have to spend a lot of time doing a lot of exercises in order to get stronger and pain-free – which is simply untrue. If your exercise program is targeting the *correct* problem with *effective* exercises, then you should not be spending all day doing dozens of exercises. Of course there are exceptions, but they are few.

Another misconception is that simple, uncomplicated exercises are ineffective. Take stretching for example. Pulling your heel up to your buttock, and holding it there for a mere thirty-seconds, once a day, may appear to some readers to be too simple a maneuver, or too short a time frame to ever stretch out a tight muscle. But on the contrary, multiple randomized controlled trials have consistently pointed out that stretching for a longer period of time, or more times a day, will not produce better results.

Finally, the last common misconception deals with not trying an exercise because, "I've done that one before and it didn't help." The interesting thing I've noted is that when you question someone carefully about what they actually did, you often find that while a person may in fact have been doing an exercise correctly, they have *not* been following proper evidence-based guidelines. Using stretching as an example again, let's say that a person tries a particular stretch that is indeed targeting the correct tight muscle, only they've been holding the stretch for fifteen-seconds, instead of the proven thirty-seconds.

After getting poor results for a period of time, most people will usually abandon the exercise and think, "That stretch didn't work." The truth, however, is that they really were doing a helpful exercise, it's just that they weren't following the correct evidence-based guidelines to make the exercise effective.

The moral? When proceeding with **THE BULLETPROOF KNEE PROGRAM**, make sure that you do the exercises *exactly* as instructed, even if you've tried some of them before, or they seem too simple to be effective. Then and only then can you say with certainty that the exercises in this book were really useful or not.

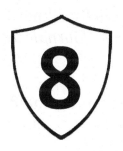

COMPREHENSIVE LIST OF SUPPORTING REFERENCES

It's true! All the information in this book is based on randomized controlled trials and scientific studies that have been published in peer-reviewed journals. Since I know there are readers out there like myself that like to actually check out the information for themselves, I've included the references for *every* study I have cited in this book. Never trust a self-help book that doesn't have sound research to support its advice...

CHAPTER 1

Bhattacharyya T, et al. The clinical importance of meniscal tears demonstrated by magnetic resonance imaging in osteoarthritis of the knee. *Journal of Bone and Joint Surgery* 2007;85-A:4-9.

Eastlack M, et al. Laxity, instability, and functional outcome after ACL injury: copers versus noncopers. *Medicine and Science in Sports and Exercise* 1999;31:210-215.

Eitzen I, et al. Anterior cruciate ligament-deficient potential copers and noncopers reveal different isokinetic quadriceps strength profiles in the early stage after injury. *The American Journal of Sports Medicine* 2010;38:586-593.

Hannan M, et al. Analysis of the discordance between radiographic changes and knee pain in osteoarthritis of the knee. *J Rheumatology* 2000;27:1513-1517.

Johnson L, et al. Clinical assessment of asymptomatic knees: comparison of men and women. *Arthroscopy: The Journal of Arthroscopic and Related Surgery* 1998;14:347-359.

Kaplan Y. Identifying individuals with an anterior cruciate ligament-deficient knee as copers and noncopers: a narrative review. *Journal of Orthopaedic and Sports Physical Therapy* 2011;41:758-766.

Zanetti M, et al. Patients with suspected meniscal tears: prevalence of abnormalities seen on MRI of 100 symptomatic and 100 contralateral asymptomatic knees. *AJR* 2003;181:635-641.

CHAPTER 3

Ageberg E, et al. 15-year follow-up of neuromuscular function in patients with unilateral nonreconstructed anterior cruciate ligament injury initially treated with rehabilitation and activity modification. *The American Journal of Sports Medicine* 2007;35:2109-2117.

Al-Hourani K, et al. Recovery of knee function in the isolated MCL and combined ACL-MCL deficient knee. *Journal of Clinical Orthopaedics and Trauma* 2015;6:89-93.

Berger R, et. al. Effect of various repetitive rates in weight training on improvements in strength and endurance. *J Assoc Phys Mental Rehabil* 1966;20:205-207.

Braith R, et. al. Comparison of 2 vs 3 days/week of variable resistance training during 10- and 18- week programs. *Int J Sports Med* 1989;10:450-454.

Carolan B, Cafarelli E. Adaptations in coactivation after isometric resistance training. *J Appl Physiol* 1992;73:911-917.

Carroll T, et. al. Resistance training frequency: strength and myosin heavy chain responses to two and three bouts per week. *Eur J Appl Physiol* 1998;78:270-275.

DeMichele P, et. al. Isometric torso rotation strength: effect of training frequency on its development. *Arch Phys Med Rehabil* 1997;78:64-69.

Esquivel A, et al. High and low volume resistance training and vascular function. *Int J of Sports Med* 2007;28:217-221.

Fahrer H, et al. Knee effusion and reflex inhibition of the quadriceps. *The Journal of Bone and Joint Surgery* 1988;70-B:635-638.

Garfinkel S, Cafarelli E. Relative changes in maximal force, EMG, and muscle cross-sectional area after isometric training. *Medicine and Science in Sports and Exercise* 1992;24:1220-1227.

Hass C, et. al. Single versus multiple sets in long-term recreational weightlifters. *Medicine and Science in Sports and Exercise* 2000;32:235-242.

Hurley M, et al. The influence of arthrogenous muscle inhibition on quadriceps rehabilitiation of patients with early, unilateral, osteoarthritic knees. *British Journal of Rheumatology* 1993;32:127-131.

Hsiao S, et al. Changes of muscle mechanics associated with anterior cruciate ligament deficiency and reconstruction. *Journal of Strength and Conditioning Research* 2014;28:390-400.

Jensen K, et al. The effects of knee effusion on quadriceps strength and knee intraarticular pressure. *Arthroscopy: The Journal of Arthroscopic and Related Surgery* 1993;9:52-56.

Kannus P. Long-term results of conservatively treated medial collateral ligament injuries of the knee joint. *Clinical Orthopaedics and Related Research* 1988;226:103-112.

Kaya D, et al. Women with patellofemoral pain syndrome have quadriceps femoris volume and strength deficiency. *Knee Surg Sports Traumatol Arthrosc* 2011;19:242-247.

Lee D, et al. Quadriceps strength and endurance after posterior cruciate ligament tears versus matched group with anterior cruciate ligament tears. *Arthroscopy: The Journal of Arthroscopic and Related Surgery* 2015;31:1097-1101.

Liikavainio T, et al. Physical function and properties of quadriceps femoris muscle in men with knee osteoarthritis. *Arch Phys Med Rehabil* 2008;89:2185-94.

Manal T, et al. Failure of voluntary activation of the quadriceps femoris muscle after patellar contusion. *Journal of Orthopaedic and Sports Physical Therapy* 2000;30:654-663.

Oiestad B, et al. Knee extensor muscle weakness is a risk factor for development of knee osteoarthritis. A systematic review and meta-analysis. *Osteoarthritis and Cartilage* 2015;23:171-177.

O'Shea P. Effects of selected weight training programs on the development of strength and muscle hypertrophy. *Research Quarterly* 1966;37:95-102.

Palmieri G. Weight training and repetition speed. *Journal of Applied Sport Science Research* 1987;1:36-38.

Palmieri-Smith R, et al. Pain and effusion and quadriceps activation and strength. *Journal of Athletic Training* 2013;48:186-191.

Pattyn E, et al. Vastus medialis obliquus atrophy. Does it exist in patellofemoral pain syndrome? *The American Journal of Sports Medicine* 2011;39:1450-1455.

Reid C, et. al. Weight training and strength, cardiorespiratory functioning and body composition of men. *Br J Sports Med* 1987;21:40-44.

Silvester L, et. al. The effect of variable resistance and free-weight training programs on strength and vertical jump. *Natl Strength Cond J* 1982;3:30-33.

Slemenda C, et al. Quadriceps weakness and osteoarthritis of the knee. *Annals of Internal Medicine* 1997;127:97-104.

Spencer, J et al. Knee joint effusion and quadriceps reflex inhibition in man. *Arch Phys Med Rehabil* 1984;65:171-177.

Starkey D, et. al. Effect of resistance training volume on strength and muscle thickness. *Medicine and Science in Sports and Exercise* 1996;28:1311-1320.

Stowers T, et. al. The short-term effects of three different strength-power training methods. *Natl Strength Cond J* 1983;5:24-27.

Tibone J, et al. Functional analysis of untreated and reconstructed posterior cruciate ligament injuries. *The American Journal of Sports Medicine* 1988;16:217-223.

Young A, et al. Measurement of quadriceps muscle wasting by ultrasonography. *Rheumatology and Rehabilitation* 1980;19:141-148.

Young W, Bilby G. The effect of voluntary effort to influence speed of contraction on strength, muscular power, and hypertrophy development. *J of Strength and Conditioning Research* 1993;7:172-178.

CHAPTER 4

Ferber R, et al. Changes in knee biomechanics after hip-abductor strengthening protocol for runners with patellofemoral pain syndrome. *Journal of Athletic Training* 2011;46:142-149.

Fredericson M, et al. Hip abductor weakness in distance runners with iliotibial band syndrome. *Clinical Journal of Sports Medicine* 2000:10:169-175.

Khayambashi K, et al. The effects of isolated hip abductor and external rotator muscle strengthening on pain, health status, and hip strength in females with patellofemoral pain: a randomized controlled trial. *Journal of Orthopaedic and Sports Physical Therapy* 2012;42:22-29.

Snyder K, et al. Resistance training is accompanied by increases in hip strength and changes in lower extremity biomechanics during running. *Clinical Biomechanics* 2009;24:26-34.

Sled E, et al. Effect of a home program of hip abductor exercises on knee joint loading, strength, function, and pain in people with knee osteoarthritis: a clinical trial. *Physical Therapy* 2010;90:895-904.

CHAPTER 5

American Academy of Orthopedic Surgeons. *Joint Motion: Method of Measuring and Recording.* Chicago: AAOS, 1965.

Bandy W, Irion J. The effect of time on static stretch on the flexibility of the hamstring muscles. *Physical Therapy* 1994;74:845-852.

Bandy W, et. al. The effect of time and frequency of static stretching on flexibility of the hamstring muscles. *Physical Therapy* 1997;77:1090-1096.

Bandy W, et. al. The effect of static stretch and dynamic range of motion training on the flexibility of the hamstring muscles. *Journal of Orthopaedic and Sports Physical Therapy* 1998;27:295-300.

Clark, W.A. *"A System of Joint Measurement." J Orthop Surg* 1920;2:687.

Daniels, L., and Worthingham, C. *Muscle Testing: Techniques of Manual Examination*, 3rd ed. Philadelphia, WB Saunders: 1972.

Davis D, et al. The effectiveness of 3 stretching techniques on hamstring flexibility using consistent stretching parameters. *Journal of Strength and Conditioning Research* 2005;19:27-32.

Journal of the American Medical Association: A Guide to the Evaluation of Permanent Impairment of the Extremities and Back (special ed.) 1 1958.

Kapandji, I.A. *Physiology of the Joints*, vols 1 and 2, 2nd ed. London: Churchill Livingstone, 1970.

Kendall, F.P., and McCreary, E.K. *Muscles: Testing and Function*, 3rd ed. Baltimore: Williams and Wilkins, 1983.

Rowe, P, et al. Knee joint kinematics in gait and other functional activities measured using flexible electrogoniometry: how much knee motion is sufficient for normal daily life? *Gait and Posture* 2000;12:143-155.

CHAPTER 6

Rudolph K, et al. Dynamic stability in the anterior cruciate ligament deficient knee. *Knee Surg Sports Traumatol Arthrosc* 2001;9:62-71.

Fitzgerald G, et al. The efficacy of perturbation training in nonoperative anterior cruciate ligament rehabilitation programs for physically active individuals. *Physical Therapy* 2000;80:128-140.

Chmielewski T, et al. Perturbation training improves knee kinematics and reduces muscle co-contraction after complete unilateral anterior cruciate ligament rupture. *Physical Therapy* 2005;85:740-754.

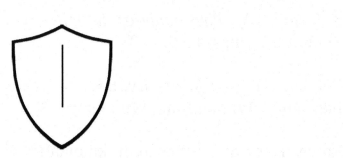

Lightning Source UK Ltd.
Milton Keynes UK
UKOW05f2147121217
314364UK00010B/562/P